Autonomy
Taking Control of Your Healthcare in a Broken System

Joseph Radich

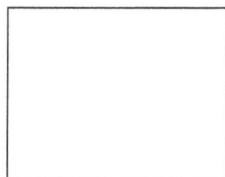

Copyright ©2022 by R3 Health Network

Cover by
Interior illustrations by Kerry Ulysse, Creative Director at R3 Health Network and Ashley Corso, Director of Research & Development at R3 Health Network

ebook ISBN: 978-8-9854025-2-0
Paperback ISBN: 978-8-9854025-7-5
Hardback ISBN: 978-8-9854025-9-9

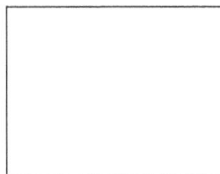

Dedication

This book has been a passion project of mine and something I have always wanted to do since I started my career in healthcare. Once I began clinical practice I quickly was exposed to the 'ugly' side and the business 'real world' of medicine which could not have been any further from what I thought I was getting myself into. This book is a culmination of 10 years' worth of trials, tribulations, late nights, early mornings, difficult conversations, joyous moments and everything in between.

The goal of this book was to open the worlds eyes and raise awareness to inconsistencies and weaknesses of our healthcare system, educate people as to why the system is what it is, speak on why the system never gets better, and what we can do as a society to help each other live healthier, longer, and more fulfilled lives.

I would like to dedicate this book to YOU, the reader, I commend you on your willingness to learn and be open minded. I hope after you have read this book, you will be more educated on ways to help yourself and those around you be better physically, mentally, emotionally, and even spiritually.

I also would like to dedicate this book to my wife Nicole, and my two girls Gabriella and Mila. Nicole, you are my shining light, my words of wisdom, my voice of reasoning, my ultimate supporter and best critic, there will never be enough words to rely what you mean to me. Without you three leading ladies in my life, my life would have an empty void and be unfulfilled.

I also must acknowledge my team and my colleagues and everyone that has ever offered me a helping hand. I would be no-where near where I am today without the help, support, and guidance of too many people to thank individually! A special thank you must go out to a few people that helped this book come to life, John, Ashley, and Kerry, thank you for all your help, hard work and dedication to me and helping me spread my voice. You all have been a blessing.

Remember, only you know your body best, so give yourself the tools you need to help yourself live your best life. Don't settle, challenge yourself and your health care practitioners. Demand answers, explanations, and the best. Surround yourself with people that believe and listen to you and who support your journey.

To your amazing health and future endeavors.

Joseph Radich

Contents

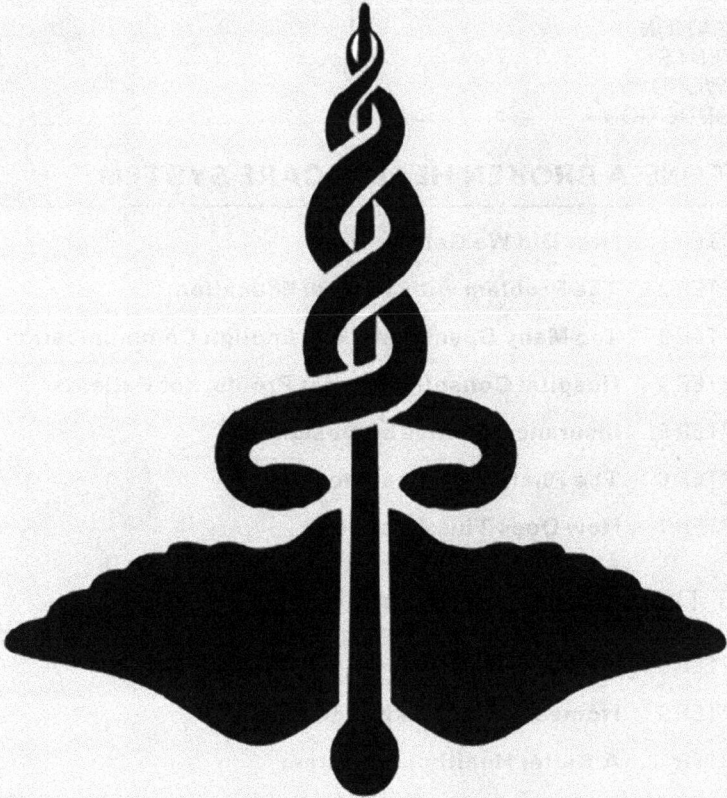

"Once we see what we (as a society) are doing or have been doing, you also see its futility, and that unconscious pattern then comes to an end by itself. Awareness is the greatest agent for change."

—Eckhart Tolle.

In order to grow and evolve we must first be self aware as to our faults.... We must recognize the upside down medical system as it stands now and be the catalyst for its change

Ever wonder what makes a great healthcare practitioner? These days there seems to be an objective list of what makes a great medical practitioner. Item one, attend a prestigious medical program. Item two, graduate at the top of your class from said prestigious program. Item three, study under someone who has been working in your field of interest for many years who has also completed items one and two. However, being a great healthcare provider is more subjective than you'd think. But all those things sometimes don't translate into good healthcare practice. There are many intelligent and intellectual people on this planet, but not everyone can be an excellent health care practitioner. A great healthcare practitioner possesses certain innate characteristics and personality trats that cannot be taught or learned by some medical textbook or prestigious medical school curriculum. These innate characteristics are what separate good healthcare practitioners from great healthcare practitioners. Throughout this book, we will highlight four innate qualities that select few health care practitioners possess.

Empathy

Compassion

Genuine

Teacher

Think about these qualities and reflect on your relationship with your current healthcare provider. If they don't embody these characteristics of a great healer, chances are you are falling victim to our broken system. As you pursue your health journey through life, be sure that you surround yourself with people that possess these qualities, as they will offer you insights and support that is invaluable.

Foreword

A flashbulb memory is a phenomenon in which a vivid recollection of a consequential life event lives on exactly as it happened, in your brain forever. I had just gotten home from aftercare; I was in the fifth grade. I noticed my healthy, active father appear as white as a sheet and sweating as if he had just been working out. My mom rushed me into my brother's room and within 5-minutes ambulances filled the street and paramedics rushed into our home. Not aware at the time, my dad was having a massive heart attack and this was a moment that would shape the rest of my life.

From the age of 10 onward, I have experienced the workings of the United States Healthcare system in most all capacities. My father was bounced around from specialist to specialist trying to figure out what was triggering his worsening congestive heart failure. He received emergency care, hospitalized cardiac care, and a very long stay in the intensive care unit that finally resulted in a heart transplant. I have experienced post-transplant care and again the bouncing around from specialists to manage the symptoms of anti-rejection medications.

Dealing with all these facets of healthcare for so long, I was able to observe the vital healthcare workers in all their many different roles. They always seemed tired, overworked, and generally unhappy. Like all kids who take a liking to science, I was sure I wanted to be a doctor when I grew up. However, the more experience I had in medical settings the more I realized I needed to do something different. I aspired to work with science and patients, but most importantly I sought to have the opportunity to truly make a difference in patient's lives.

Freshly out of college I had the pleasure of meeting the author of this book, Joseph Radich. I was bright eyed and bushy-tailed and ready to put my passion for biochemistry to work. I took a job with a cutting-edge business, promising to deliver regenerative therapies to help patients suffering from chronic diseases like congestive heart failure. Through this company, I felt I would be able to truly make a difference in the lives of people who were just like me, desperate to help their loved ones get better.

My time with this company did not prove to be all that I once thought it would be. I was passionate about the work and the mission, but the goals always seemed to get lost by way of big egos. I noticed patterns of behavior that I saw frequently in the traditional hospital settings. The boss was always right (*even if they weren't*); there was no collaboration amongst medical providers and patients on the best treatment plan. I found myself displaying behaviors that I had seen for years, all stemming from being generally unhappy with my role in healthcare. In the end, the leaders of the organization lost sight of the mission and their ego's drove the company into the ground, which just might have been the best thing to happen to me.

I began working full time for one of the greatest healthcare providers I have ever had the pleasure of knowing, Joseph Radich. When I first met Joe several years before working for him, he told me that we were going to change the way that healthcare is delivered in this world. This is a statement I find myself reflecting on a lot, even to this day. Joe has followed through with this mission. He has created an environment that ensures all decisions are based in groundbreaking scientific discoveries and tailored to individuals' biochemistry. More important than that, he ensures all patients are involved in their healthcare. Joe takes the time to educate patients, provide them with tools necessary for lifestyle changes, and consistently follows up- not just when they're sick. Joe has taught me that patients are not names on charts- they are people who we have the pleasure of helping.

I trust that this book will educate its readers on the core values of what makes an exceptional healthcare provider. The same values that Joe has instilled in me throughout my young professional career.

Ashley Corso
Director of Research and Development at R3 Health Network

Introduction

What Can this Book Do for You?

The year 2020 will be remembered as one of the most challenging years in modern U.S. history. The country was ravaged by the coronavirus, suffering through waves of infection that closed down much of the country for months at a time and resulted in more than half a million people dying from COVID-19.

Throughout the pandemic, tensions ran high—we all were on edge. Stressed by the pandemic, many people suffered from anxiety and depression, and millions of people turned to poor health decisions as a coping mechanism or just purely to get through it. As a country, we ate more, exercised less, skipped seeing the doctor, slept less, and otherwise made even more negative lifestyle choices. The effect of the pandemic will be felt in our bodies, our minds, our wallets, our spirits, and in many more unfathomable ways for years to come, both here in the United States and throughout the world. Never have we seen such a devastating and life-altering phenomena throughout the world!

Alongside the grim personal reality of living through COVID-19, the pandemic will also be remembered for laying bare the problems with the U.S. medical system. Problems that had long plagued our system were brutally exposed as the United States—supposedly the most technically and medically advanced country in the world—quickly led the world in pandemic-related complications and deaths. Our hospitals experienced shortages of basic medical equipment and staff, plus lack of medications to treat the virus. At the same time, medical and statistical misinformation ran rampant through the population as people turned to misguided therapies, conflicting medical advice, and didn't know who to listen to, what and who to believe, and what to do. Making matters even worse, we suffered through arguably the most controversial political and social time in our country's history, with diametrically opposed medical messaging from both ends of the political spectrum and news media outlets. The media quickly filled with stories of surprise medical outcomes and bills for COVID-19 patients, as many patients received bills for tens or even hundreds of thousands of dollars. These horror stories further froze people in place, leading many to take no action at all, which quickly led to the worsening of the pandemic.

The failure of our system shocked much of the country, along with most of the world. But it shouldn't have. The issues that crippled the U.S. response to the pandemic have long been obvious to those of us who try to work within America's creaking medical system. Inequality in care, lack of consistency, lack of continuity of care, lack of resources, surprise medical bills (influence from insurance carriers), and a poor record delivering preventative care have been basic features of the U.S. medical system for decades now.

While the idea for this book came long before the pandemic, COVID-19 turned out to be the tragic straw that broke the camel's back. It focused all of the reasons why I wanted to write this book and why we all need to hear this message. We can't let the circumstances and lessons to be learned of 2020 slip into the rearview mirror in our hurry to get our "normal" lives back. The fact is, when it comes to the U.S. medical system, the "normal" system was already failing us. The pandemic is just the dramatic climax to a movie that has been playing for years, a movie that depicts one of the world's most powerful country's failing medical system and its deep-rooted corruption. Everything from our medical schools to our insurance and hospital industries and even the Internet have conspired to confuse Americans, making us sicker, broker, and more skeptical than ever before.

This book is my attempt to address the shortcomings in the U.S. medical system, to raise awareness about why the healthcare system has gotten so out of control. My goal is to raise awareness and show how people can navigate a broken system to ensure that their health is a top priority. In my clinics, we are pioneering and mastering a new approach to medicine. Our core values and unique approach make it possible for us to deliver high-quality care that makes a real difference in our patients' lives. We listen to our patients; we get to know our patients. We build lifelong relationships with our patients. Our approach focuses on prophylactic disease prevention and health optimization rather than reactive disease management. We strive to educate our patients on why their bodies do what they do and teach our patients what they need to know to live the highest quality of life for the longest period of time. We practice true anti-aging medicine!

Our approach is driven by advances across medicine, both traditional medicine and the so-called "alternative" practices, and we know it works.

We call our combination approach "integrative and regenerative medicine." I've seen tens of thousands of patients turn their lives around by changing the way they think about their own health and then taking action. In medical schools we are taught the concept of "autonomy," meaning the privilege of self–decision making. As individuals, we are blessed with many important civil liberties; however, the right to medical self-decision has fallen victim to our poorly functioning healthcare system. Too many people have lost autonomy in their health journey.

Now more than ever, patients are told what to do and when/how to do it. Patients aren't given the information they need to make their own decisions. Without restoring medical autonomy, our healthcare system will never get better. In this book, my primary objective is to raise awareness about *why* we have lost our medical autonomy, *what* drives this poor healthcare system, and *how* we can improve our healthcare system. I'm proposing a new way of thinking about medicine and health.

There has never been a better time for a book like this. I firmly believe the only way to improve our healthcare system is to ignite a patient-driven revolution in medicine. And believe me when I tell you that spark has been lit—the patients who come to our clinics are at the leading edge of this revolution. Our patients don't just believe "doctor knows best." Instead, they have researched their conditions and want to understand them. Many of these individuals have had bad experiences or experienced failed conventional therapies and practitioners, or they are just simply looking to learn and understand their bodies better. They are ready for a better, more integrated, whole-body approach to healthcare that helps them actually look and feel their best—and live their best lives. They ask tough questions, challenge their healthcare providers, and they take the time to learn what they need to know to protect their health and slow or even reverse aging.

Our time on this planet is short, and we want to help make sure that you live the best life you can for the longest period of time. This is true health optimization. Unfortunately, I believe unless you break from our current health care system, you will never achieve health optimization.

My patients inspire me. I look forward to communicating with our patients, as I often learn just as much from them as they from me. Our bodies are amazingly complex organisms, with hundreds of millions of cells completing hundreds of millions of reactions simultaneously to maintain internal balance (homeostasis) and promote health. Like a symphony orchestra, all of our body's cells and organ systems must work together in order to ensure and maintain glowing, vibrant health from the inside out. It's long past time to switch our mindset from disease being a sick organ or natural side effect of aging that requires intervention with a knife or pill to taking control of our own bodies and our personal medical and health journeys. It's time to change the mindset of the healthcare industry so people can take control of their own health and restore their autonomy.

We have a long way to go to make this radical change and shift a very stubborn old-school train of thought—I get that. But that's no excuse. On any given week I spend hours and hours on the phone, trying to convince conventionally practicing practitioners not to scare their patients away from integrative therapies that are proven to work. This dynamic under-lies one of the biggest barriers to a true medical revolution. Patients are confused. They're hearing different things from different practitioners, and quite often these two vantage points are completely opposite. So, what does a patient do? They do nothing, and thus no change is ever made by you or the patient, and they continue to live their lives in the ever long-ing "hamster wheel" of poor health, unhealthy lifestyle and aging because they have not been made aware of what catalyst they need to spark change. We need to open the lines of communication between practitioners—all healthcare providers should have the same goal in mind: improving the health and well-being of our patients. Unfortunately, this concept is often neglected, as specialties don't communicate effectively (if at all) with other specialties or even patients' "primary care" providers (who are supposed to be the medical quarterback for you; or even worse so, some practitioners' egos get in the way and close-mindedness and older medical teachings remain president, and yet again there is no catalyst to induce a change for the patient. The result? Back into the "hamster wheel." I've heard countless stories from women who have been scared away from effective hormone therapy, or patients who have been put on serious pharmaceuticals with-out a second thought and little education. I've watched too many patients undergo procedures they weren't prepared for, only to have traumatic and terrible outcomes.

But as a healthcare provider and a physician-trainer, I also see that the tide is changing. More and more patients are like ours: empowered, knowledgeable, not afraid to push back against bad advice and challenge their healthcare givers. New therapies are constantly being introduced and pushed by innovative clinics like ours. Even the creaking old medical industry, with its networks of overpriced medical schools, flush corpora-tions, and hospital networks, is starting to move in the right direction. In the future, I'm firmly convinced we're going to see a new kind of patient emerge, one who is in control of their own healthcare decisions and works in a true partnership with their healthcare providers. This is how medicine needs to be practiced in order to yield the best outcomes. We need to strive for individuals who have the knowledge and tools to be truly autonomous. These individuals already exist; they are thirsting for the knowledge, support, and guidance, as they know conventional healthcare is a mess, and they're banging on the door. All we need to do is help them open it.

PART ONE
A BROKEN HEALTHCARE SYSTEM

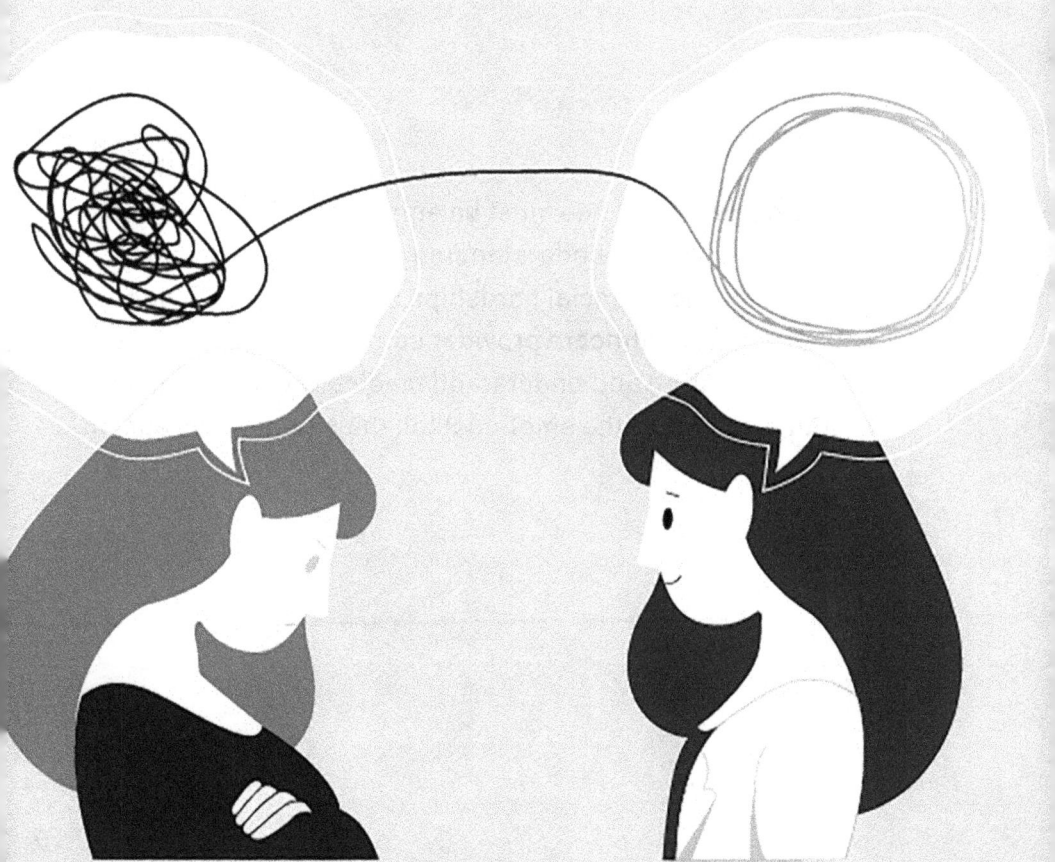
EMPATHY

To be a good healer, one must be empathetic. This involves having a cognitive understanding of patients physical, emotional, and financial hardships and feeling. By being empathetic, a healthcare provider can put themselves in a patient's position and understand medically what is taking place, but also gather the emotional toll the situation is causing.

Chapter 1

How Did We Get Here?

"If one day you find that you do not love your work, do not love your patients, have lost all hope—you must first find yourself again. How can a hopeless doctor give hope to patients? If you feel trapped, if you feel like a victim, then you are teaching your patients (and the next generation of physicians) to be victims too. Doctor means teacher."

—Pamela L. Wible, MD

The industry of medicine is in a crisis. It's plagued by high costs and distrust among the very people it was meant to serve: the patients. You and me. People are sick of the high costs and hidden medical bills. They are confused by the conflicting messages coming from various medical authorities. And they feel neglected by the one-size-fits-all, assembly-line approach to medicine they experience everywhere from private clinics to elite hospitals.

But it wasn't always like this.

In today's byzantine, expensive, and glacially slow medical "industry," it can be hard to imagine how innovation used to happen. Before medicine was turned into a profit-making enterprise for an ever-smaller group of corporations, medical innovation was often the result of a single enterprising doctor or inventor with an idea. They worked on their own, sometimes experimenting on themselves—like catheterization pioneer Charles Gruentzig did when he catheterized his own heart under X-ray to prove his heart wouldn't explode if a catheter was introduced into it.

Despite his discovery of a device that would revolutionize cardiac medicine, Gruentzig was mocked when the world learned of his experiments. Other doctors considered him crazy, and the "real" surgeons of the day dismissed his homemade catheters as useless trinkets at best and deadly distractions at worst.

And Gruentzig was far from alone. In fact, throughout history, doctors and innovators who pushed against medical knowledge were routinely attacked and sometimes driven from medicine. Perhaps the best example of this is Dr. Ignaz Semmelweis. Dr. Semmelweis was a Hungarian doctor who practiced medicine in Vienna in the first half of the 19th century.

Shortly after earning his doctorate in medicine, Dr. Semmelweis was appointed assistant in the First Obstetrical Clinic at the Vienna General Hospital. At the time, the First Obstetrical Clinic had a maternal mortality rate between 10 and 20 percent, making it one of the most dangerous places in Vienna to have a baby. Dr. Semmelweis made it his mission to understand why this was happening.

Back in those days, especially in teaching hospitals like the Vienna General Hospital, it was common for medical students to travel freely between wards, including the morgue. Dr. Semmelweis hypothesized that medical students were transmitting "cadaveric" agents to new mothers as a result of doing autopsies, then going straight into the birthing wards and working with new mothers. His proposed solution? Washing hands. It was that simple.

But it really wasn't—not for his time. In the mid-1800s in continental Europe, the "germ theory" of disease was not yet widely accepted, so the idea that an invisible killer could be transmitted from corpses to laboring mothers was considered outlandish and impossible. Nevertheless, Dr. Semmelweis instituted a new policy: all students and physicians would have to wash their hands between handling cadavers and working with living patients.

It didn't take long for Dr. Semmelweis to quickly be proven right. As a result of his new handwashing policy, the maternal mortality rate dropped to 1 to 2 percent.

You would think Dr. Semmelweis would be recognized for this staggering improvement in patient care. But that's not what happened. Instead, Dr. Semmelweis's colleagues felt he was laying blame for dead new mothers at their feet, and they rebelled against him. Doctors actually refused to wash their hands to make a point, and the political forces at his hospital lined up against him. Dr. Semmelweis would eventually be forced from the hospital and from medicine entirely. He suffered a breakdown and was committed to an asylum, where he died within a month.*

One of the problems Dr. Semmelweis faced was his inability to explain exactly why handwashing helped stop the spread of disease. It wasn't until twenty years later that another much more familiar pioneer, Louis Pasteur, confirmed the so-called "germ theory" of disease and the medical world soon followed.

It would be almost impossible to put a timestamp on the exact moment modern medicine began, but there are a few singular leaps forward that stand out. Pasteur's work is one of these leaps forward, but it might be fair to say that a pair of discoveries benefited human health more than any other advances: the development of vaccines to prevent viral diseases, and the development of antibiotics to treat bacterial diseases. Together, these twin advances—which actually happened more than a century apart, even though their mass adoption would happen nearly simultaneously in the 20th century—did more to improve human health than almost any other innovations before or since.

At the time, viral diseases had been among humankind's most feared killers for thousands of years. Long before we knew what viruses were, people lived in fear of the death and damage they caused. Smallpox—a disease we hardly even think about in today's developed world—was one of the most feared diseases in human history. It appears in ancient writings both in Egypt and China, long before the birth of Christ. Smallpox had an average mortality rate of about 30 percent and often left survivors disfigured.

By the late 18th century, however, it was suspected that giving someone a small dose of infected fluid from a smallpox sore or a similar pox could somehow protect them against the disease. This is exactly the theory of modern vaccination, and although the practice (known as variolation) was known in antiquity, it wasn't until 1796 that an English physician named Edward Jenner proved that vaccination worked. To prove it, he took a small sample of cowpox from a milk maid named Sarah Nelmes and used it to inoculate the nine-year-old son of his gardener, a boy named James Phipps. After letting a few months pass, Dr. Jenner later challenged James's

---

* Wikipedia. "Ignaz Semmelweis." https://en.wikipedia.org/wiki/Ignaz_Semmelweis.

immunity with multiple direct exposures to smallpox. The boy never developed the disease, and the age of vaccination was launched.*

As frightening as viral diseases like smallpox, tuberculosis, and the flu were, they had lethal competition: bacterial infection. Three of history's most lethal killers are bacterium, including:

- The Black Plague, also known as the bubonic plague, which wiped out a quarter of Europe's population in the 14th century.†

- Cholera, which caused a series of deadly pandemics in the 18thcentury that killed tens of millions.‡

- Tuberculosis, which killed one out of seven people in the United States at the time of its discovery in 1882.§

Like viruses, bacteria were poorly understood. The first bacteria were observed by Antonie van Leeuwenhoek in 1676, hundreds of years before humanity understood what we were looking at. It would be another two centuries before Louis Pasteur proved his germ theory, and another fifty years beyond that until yet another pioneering doctor named Alexander Fleming noticed something odd about a culture sample in his lab at St. Mary's Hospital in London.

Dr. Fleming spent World War I in the army, where he watched many of his fellow soldiers dying not from bullet wounds, but from infections that set in after the initial wound. After the war ended, he launched his research career looking for agents that could kill these infectious microorganisms. In 1928, he was working with a common staphylococcal bacteria when he noticed something odd: bacteria were dying in one particular petri dish. This dish was located next to an open window and had been inoculated with mold. Fleming isolated the type of mold and identified it as a *Penicillium* mold, then hypothesized that some kind of "mold juice" was killing bacteria. He named this mold juice "penicillin" and soon learned it was effective against all gram-positive bacteria. This fearsome list included diseases like scarlet fever, pneumonia, meningitis, and diphtheria.

---

* Woolhouse M, Scott F, Hudson Z, Howey R, Chase-Topping M. Human viruses: discovery and emergence. *Philos Trans R Soc Lond B Biol Sci.* 2012;367(1604):2864-2871. doi:10.1098/rstb.2011.0354.

† Wikipedia. "Black Death." https://en.wikipedia.org/wiki/Black_Death.

‡ The College of Physicians of Philadelphia. The history of vaccines, https://www.historyofvaccines.org/timeline#EVT_102205.

§ Centers for Disease Control and Prevention. History of World TB Day. https://www.cdc.gov/tb/worldtbday/history.htm.

Fleming published his paper on the world's first antibiotic in 1929, but the publication was met mostly with indifference. Moreover, Fleming himself had trouble producing large quantities of penicillin, so he was reduced to sending around samples of his precious mold to see if anyone could figure out how to extract it. It wasn't until the 1940s, after World War II had started and there was dire need for antibiotics, that a partnership between industry and government finally figured out how to mass-produce penicillin through fermentation. Penicillin not only protected injured Allied troops from infection, its production represented the founding of the modern pharmaceutical industry. After the war, American companies rapidly expanded around the world, opening plants to produce penicillin in dozens of countries and launching efforts to discover new antibiotics.* For his chance discovery, Dr. Alexander Fleming was awarded the Nobel Prize in 1945.

By the 1950s, with vaccine development taking off (including the introduction of the polio vaccine, which boosted vaccines' credibility as it eliminated a disease that families lived in fear of), there were rapid advances throughout medicine. In a few short decades, modern bypass surgery and minimally invasive surgery was introduced. Transplant procedures were developed and then mastered, making it possible to perform human-to-human heart and heart and lung transplants.

Thanks to improved medicine and nutrition, human life expectancy began to increase rapidly. In 1900, the average human life expectancy in the United States was 48 years old. From there, it jumped to 67 years old by 1950, on its way to 78.94 years old by 2015.†

The Deadly Consequences of Innovation Stagnation

These are inspiring stories, but what do they have to do with today? We already have antibiotics and vaccines. We understand the importance of infection control in hospitals. And we have more tools than ever before to live long, healthy lives.

Right?

Unfortunately, not so fast. Life expectancy in the United States in the past century has only dropped twice. The first time was during the Spanish

---

* Tan SY, Tatsumura Y. Alexander Fleming (1881-1955): Discoverer of penicillin. *Singapore Med J.* 2015;56(7):366-367. doi:10.11622/smedj.2015105.
† Statista. Life expectancy (from birth) in the United States, from 1860 to 2020. https://www.statista.com/statistics/1040079/life-expectancy-united-states-all-time/.

Medical Milestones

Vaccines and antibiotics were key developments for human health—but they aren't the only medical advances to improve human health. Here are some of the key innovations throughout medical history:

1846: William T. Morton introduces the use of ether during surgery as an anesthetic.

1895: The X-ray is invented by Wilhelm Conrad Röntgen.

1914: The electrocardiograph is introduced in the United States.

1922: Insulin becomes available in the United States.

1945: The Pap smear is introduced to detect cervical cancer.

1950: The first study declaring smoking a health risk is published in JAMA.

1954: The first successful kidney transplant is performed in Boston. Oral contraceptives are introduced.

1955: Ultrasound is introduced as a medical imaging tool.

1963: The first lung transplant is performed.

1964: Doctors at Mass General figure out how to store human blood for the long-term.

1967: The first heart transplant is performed.

1973: Magnetic resonance imagery is introduced.

1982: Telomeres are discovered.

1991: The first cancer vaccine is invented (but not FDA-approved until 2010).

1995: The first triple-organ (two lungs and a heart) transplant is performed.

---

flu pandemic in 1918, when it dropped sharply but then rebounded. And the second drop in life expectancy is happening right now—even without factoring in the lethal effects of the 2020 COVID-19 pandemic. In fact, American life expectancy has been dropping steadily for years. This is happening despite the United States having the most advanced medical technology in the world, the most sophisticated system of funding medical innovation in the world, and many of the world's top medical schools. For many observers, it's almost impossible to believe how poor our medical outcomes are.

But it's true. We are a nation of sick, overweight, stressed, and indebted people. Consider just a few facts:

- Between 2015 and 2020, life expectancy dropped in the United States for only the second time in a century. In 2015, two economists from Princeton, Anne Case and Angus Deaton, coined a term for the afflictions behind this increase: diseases of despair. These include drug abuse, alcoholism, and suicide—all of which have skyrocketed in the past decade.*

- In 2017 to 2018, 42 percent of American adults were considered obese, an increase of almost 50 percent from 2000. This is a disaster from a public health perspective. Obesity is linked to increases in the rate of heart disease (the nation's leading killer), certain types of cancer, liver and kidney disease, hormone imbalance, and overall premature death.† The estimated annual cost of dealing with obesity and the diseases it causes is $147 billion, and that's not counting the untold billions people spend on fad diet plans and books, "diet" foods, and other potions and pills pushed by unscrupulous quacks.

- A staggering forty million Americans experience clinical anxiety every year, or 18 percent of the population. Most of those cases are never treated. At the same time, more than sixteen million Americans suffer from major depressive disorder (MDD) every year, making it the leading cause of disability in the United States for people in their prime working years.‡

- Finally, medical expenses are by far the leading cause of personal bankruptcy in the United States. According to the *American Journal of Public Health*, in 2019, 66.5 percent of all bankruptcies in the U.S. were caused by medical bills. It's well known among emergency room doctors that patients with serious injuries are often very concerned about their cost of their treatment, even while they're being treated. A single serious disease or bad accident can easily result in hundreds of thousands

---

* Forbes. "Diseases of Despair" contribute to declining U.S. life expectancy." (July 19, 2018). https://www.forbes.com/sites/joshuacohen/2018/07/19/diseases-of-despair-contribute-to-declining-u-s-life-expectancy/#4a74dfba656b.

† Centers for Disease Control and Prevention. Adult obesity facts. https://www.cdc.gov/obesity/data/adult.html.

‡ Anxiety and Depression Association of America. Facts & statistics: did you Know? https://adaa.org/about-adaa/press-room/facts-statistics?gclid=CjwKCAjwjLD4BRAiEiwAg5NBFoRP-yVPtm0cgi0mr95Dm9iuxKbw3uccnrHkZawtd3xgzFwk-7GkqxoCwG4QAvD_BwE.

of dollars in debt, wiping out retirement accounts, savings and college accounts, and even home equity. And this can happen *even if* your family has insurance.*

So how did we get here? How did we get from a healthcare system that fostered innovation and provided steadily improving results to today's dismal situation?

Our healthcare system in this country is characterized by gross inequality, inefficiency, outsized corporate and lobbying influence, over- and under-regulation, and opaque pricing practices that are literally bankrupting families. The sad truth is that if you're very wealthy, you can afford access to the best acute medical care in the world—but you'll still suffer from the systemic issues facing our healthcare system, including a top-down approach to your own health where questions are discouraged and the "doctor knows best" no matter how long he or she has been practicing and how current their knowledge is. You'll still likely be denied access to potentially lifesaving information about how to really prevent and treat chronic diseases. Instead, you'll be billed exorbitant amounts for the same substandard preventive care models that are literally killing everyone else. This isn't even to mention the fact that what most conventionally practicing practitioners consider "normal" is not, in fact, normal or even close to optimal. The wait-to-react approach toward healthcare is the primary objective whether you're wealthy or not. Even access to the "best" medical care does not guarantee it will be tailored to your body's needs and goals. And the concept of optimal health is still a mirage.

And if you aren't rich? You're on your own, left to navigate a complex world of billing codes, actuarial restrictions, stressed and overworked healthcare providers who don't have ten minutes to spend with you at a time, and eye-popping cost for basic pharmaceuticals and procedures. For most patients, there is little to no attention paid to preventing disease, and patients are overwhelmed with complex information and no sustained effort to educate them on how to practice better self-care. How many times has your doctor ever taken the time to explain how lifestyle really affects health? How much do you know about the self-inflicted issues that are literally killing us, the toxins, pollution, stress, and dietary choices that are causing our own medical demise?

---

* Investopedia. Top 5 reasons why people go bankrupt. https://www.investopedia.com/financial-edge/0310/top-5-reasons-people-go-bankrupt.aspx.

The way my schedule is built, and this the unfortunate majority of medical professionals, I have fifteen minutes for follow-up visits and thirty minutes for new patients. And they want to cut that to ten minutes and twenty minutes. It takes a lot more time than that to have a meaningful conversation.

But we're jammed up by insurance. My boss needs an excuse to continue to pay salaries, so I need to generate revenue and that means more patients. Insurance does not value quality. They value quantity.

—Evelina Grayver, MD, FACC
Director of Women's Heart Health, Northwell Central Region and Katz Women's Institute

It can be tempting to blame your doctor, but physicians themselves are stuck in the same system you are. No matter who you are, insurance tables and Medicare regulations drive most clinical choices and the way that healthcare practitioners practice. Physicians are rarely granted freedom and time to practice medicine the best way they know how. There are treatment quotas to meet and outrageous liability protection to afford, not to mention the often-crushing cost of physician student loans.

The worst thing about the situation we find ourselves in is that it wasn't an accident, and it didn't have to be like this. Rather, our current medical system is the product of a series of deliberate choices made over the course of decades by people with a lot to gain. At almost every level of the medical industry, profiteers have fought to institute government regulations and laws that hopelessly twist the system out of shape. Yet the group that's most affected—patients themselves—you and me—never have a seat at the table when these decisions are made.

In the best circumstances, we try not to think about it while we're healthy, and hope for the best if we do get sick or injured. And if you do get sick? It's virtually impossible for anyone except an expert to understand what's really going on. How many people can really break down the complex system of manufacturers, PBMs, insurance companies, and retailers that make up our pharmaceutical industry? When you pay $100 or $200 for a new prescription, do you really have any idea where that money is going?

But understanding this system is necessary if we're going to change it. And change it we must. For any number of reasons—simple fairness, an aging country, to stop the deterioration in our general health—we need to step up and make changes in what we are willing to accept from a broken healthcare system. And the first change? Like Gandhi said, we can be the change we want to see in the world. It begins with understanding what's actually happening, and then you can rebuild your own healthcare plan, one that you are in control of and that is designed to prevent you from getting an entirely preventable disease that may potentially bankrupt you and rob you of good years. It's time for a paradigm shift, and not just one that takes us back to the time when giants of medicine working in obscure labs changed the world. In the future, the world will continue to grow more connected, more technologically capable, more diverse, and with a dizzying range of options and access to information. Medicine in the future must take this future into account and hand power back to empowered consumers, back to the physicians who are motivated to treat patients and not meet quotas. And that is really the fundamental challenge in this book: arming you with information so when you look in the mirror, you are part of the solution.

Chapter 2

The Problem with Medical Education

"*The dilemma of modern medicine, and the underlying central flaw in medical education and, most of all, in the training of interns, is the irresistible drive to do something, anything. It is expected by patients and too often agreed to by their doctors, in the face of ignorance.*"

—Lewis Thomas

Let's imagine a young woman named Breanna. Breanna's in high school and has always dreamed of being a doctor. Perhaps she cared for her mother during her mother's diagnosis with breast cancer, and she saw firsthand her mother's suffering from the disease, along with her family's struggle to make sure her mom was getting the best care possible. After her mother passed away following two years of treatments that included debilitating chemotherapy, radiation therapy and surgery, Breanna vowed she would go into medicine and devote her life to helping families like her own trying to beat breast cancer.

As a high school student, Breanna is already making choices that will affect her future career in medicine. She'll need high grades and a good SAT score to get into a decent undergraduate college. But as she prepares to head off to college, the first of her compromising choices is already upon her. She can go to a cheaper, local school and save money by living at home, or she can borrow money to go to a more prestigious school. If her goal is to get into a top medical school, she'll need the transcript power of the higher-ranked undergraduate school, so she picks that school and racks up $60,000 in undergraduate debt while achieving the kind of grades that can get admission into a top medical school.

During college, she has the opportunity to shadow healthcare practitioners to gain critical and required "direct patient contact hours." It is here that Breanna starts to get a more comprehensive understanding of what "working in medicine" entails. She sees physicians attend to forty to sixty patients per day, spending less than ten minutes with each patient, followed by hours of clinical notes and charting, and countless argumentative phone calls with insurance companies and specialists. Unfortunately, surrounded by working clinicians, Breanna quickly begins to think this is "normal" and how medicine should be practiced.

After she graduates, she starts applying to medical schools—with no other option than to borrow more money to get her medical degree. In fact, by the time she graduates her four-year program from a prestigious medical school, she is hundreds of thousands of dollars in debt and heading into a residency program where she can expect to work round the clock for two years for very little pay. When she's done with her residency, she signs up for another two-year program in her specialty as a fellow with the same unfathomable work schedule for very sub-par compensation. All told, Breanna will have spent eight years in formal post-secondary schooling and four years in post-graduate residencies, racking up incredible debt, all before she actually begins to practice.

And this is where the real pressure begins. At this point, Breanna is under intense pressure to pay off her student loans and to protect herself from liability. When it comes to finding a job, the financial aspect weighs on every decision she makes. Unfortunately, what gets lost is her original reason she got into medicine in the first place: to beat breast cancer. Just like the physicians she shadowed in college, Breanna soon finds herself in a role where she has much less patient contact than she'd imagined and spends much more time on paperwork and arguing with insurance companies than she thought possible. Moreover, it quickly becomes apparent that her very expensive education left a lot out—patients are asking about nutraceuticals and cancer protocols that combine the allopathic medicine she learned so much about in school with alternative approaches. Despite all of her education, she can't answer these questions on nutrition and functional medicine. After all, across her twelve years of medical school she spent less than fifty hours talking about lifestyle medicine.

Now, Breanna is faced with the prospect of educating herself on the many different ways cancer treatment can be individualized. Rather than invest more time and more money and reduce her productivity at work (thus lowering her compensation as most physicians receive productivity bonuses), Breanna decides to forget about learning about alternative methodologies and resorts to downplaying these "alternative" treatments. Instead, she steers her patients toward more accepted models of therapy, despite the wealth of published studies on different approaches. And thus, Breanna falls victim to a very common evolution of most healthcare practitioners, and ultimately Breanna and her career will continue to escalate the problem with the healthcare industry versus her original goal to help transform the way healthcare was practiced. And this scenario happens countless of times with new medical graduates, and you can easily see why there has been no healthcare solution. As a medical professional we are conditioned to have to practice a way that is wrong, a way that violates our Hippocratic oath to "do no harm" and makes our healthcare system perpetually worse.

As a medical professional, you're no doubt familiar with some variation of this story. There are many reasons people go into medicine, but unfortunately many of those reasons quickly take a backseat to financial and administrative concerns once a soon-to-be doctor enters the academic pipeline that produces doctors. So, let's take a deeper dive into how this system lets down the very people who rely on it to work: the doctors and healthcare practitioners, who are counting on this system to provide them with the tools they need to treat patients.

Not surprisingly, the story begins with money. All college students in today's economy are facing incredible debt, but nowhere is that more pronounced than medical school. According to the American Association of Medical Colleges (AAMC), the average cost for one year at a public medical school was almost $35,000 for in-state students. This includes tuition, fees, and health insurance, but does not include housing, books, food, or any other costs. For out-of-state students, the cost averaged almost $60,000 a year. And these are public schools. For private schools, the average annual cost is in excess of $50,000.

In reality, if Breanna was to get accepted into a top medical school, it would cost much more than that. According to *US News and World Report*, the nation's most expensive medical school is Tufts University, where tuition and fees alone are $61,000 per year. The list of most expensive schools is rounded out by Ivy League schools like Columbia and Dartmouth, plus Northwestern and Case Western Reserve University.

Everyone knows college is expensive—and fortunately for thousands of families, there are lots of grants and scholarships to help fund higher education. Not so for medical education. According to the Kaplan testing company, "There are far fewer scholarships to cover the cost of medical school than are available at the undergraduate level."*

So, assuming that Breanna's parents weren't among the 1 percent, it's easy to see how she can rack up almost $200,000 in debt by the time she finally walks the stage and prepares to enter her residency. And in fact, again according to the AAMC, the median debt for med students upon graduating is $200,000—and a whopping 76 percent of medical students graduate with debt.†

Perhaps the prospect of this debt is helping to fuel the U.S.'s expected shortage of physicians. The AAMC estimates that by 2030, there will be a shortfall of almost fifty thousand primary care physicians and seventy-three thousand specialists. And who can blame the next generation for not choosing medicine after they realize that being a doctor might bring in a high salary, but it also means navigating the rigors of medical school, taking on hundreds of thousands of dollars of debt before and after thirty, and then graduating into a field where frustration, lack of freedom to practice as you see fit, and liability are the norm, not to mention the suffocating oversight many medical institutions maintain over their medical staff.

All of this might be more excusable if medical schools themselves were really delivering value to the students attending them. But they don't. Too many medical schools let our future doctors down in two very real ways.

The first is a lack of preparation for the actual world of medicine. Students are drilled on the basics—anatomy, patient presentation, disease treatment, etc.—but they aren't taught about the business of medicine. Upon graduation, they are thrust into a world far removed from the ideologically pure world of classroom medicine. They don't know how to negotiate their own contracts, and many young doctors end up signing work contracts with restrictive non-compete clauses, dictatorial administrative rules, and patient quotas. Thanks to this lack of preparation about the business of medicine, the stereotype that "doctors make the worst businesspeople" is unfortunately true. In some ways, this is good (in an ideal world, we want our healthcare providers to avoid financial bias); however, in order to practice medicine in the manner you wish, it's vital to actually

---

* Kaplan Testing. What's the real cost of medical school? https://www.kaptest.com/study/mcat/whats-the-real-cost-of-medical-school/.

† American Association of Medical Colleges. 7 Ways to Reduce Medical School Debt. https://www.aamc.org/news-insights/7-ways-reduce-medical-school-debt.

understand how the business works. Without this understanding, you'll be left at the mercy of institutions that are more than happy to dictate your every clinical decision.

As bad as this is, the second issue with medical schools is likely much worse and directly affects patient care. As I noted in the first chapter, the world of medicine is incredibly slow to adapt and change. It can take decades for something as powerful as penicillin to be recognized and mass produced. This molasses-like attitude toward change begins in medical school, where curricula are focused with laser-like intensity on a narrow band of "traditional" medical approaches and new information is viewed with suspicion and hostility. Amazingly, very few medical school curricula include any serious coursework on alternative medicine. Instead, most schools have a few courses they offer in an effort to prepare their students to debunk alternative therapies. This hostile view of alternative medical practices extends into practice, where patients who ask questions about alternative therapies are routinely shamed for asking, or they are assured that there's "insufficient evidence" a particular modality will work and it's "probably a scam" anyway.

Instead, doctors who barely understand the business of medicine are trained to use standardized clinical care paths that essentially force everyone into the same treatment modalities, suppress questions about individualized medicine, and protect the doctor and the institution they work for from liability.

Flowchart Medicine: Failing Everyone

There's so much wrong with this approach to teaching new doctors it's hard to know where to begin, but the obvious place is: with you. As a unique individual, there's no other person in the world exactly like you. If you have siblings, they're the closest, but even then there's a universe of difference between you and them. These differences aren't just genetic—you are the consequence of every choice you've ever made. How you eat. How much sleep you get. How much exercise. Do you drink alcohol or run marathons or live at high elevation. The number of factors that go into making up a human being are dizzying. Each of us is an incredibly complex chemical and mechanical system that operates with astounding precision, and each of our decisions (even the small ones) influences our physiology. People often say that our bodies are programmed to act and be a certain way, blaming subpar "genetics" for conditions like obesity. This is not the case! Although our bodies are genetically predisposed to be and act a certain way, it has been well documented that lifestyle decisions affect and change our genetic blueprint. Thus, the idea of nurture affecting nature! This is why we argue that lifestyle can overcome genetics.

Considering this, does it really make sense to assume that we'll all react the same way to the same dosage of the same medications? Of course not. For a real-world example, think about depression. Millions of Americans every year suffer from symptoms associated with a depressive disorder. This disease is common and debilitating. It costs billions of dollars a year in lost productivity and, at its worst, can rob people of their joy and even their lives. Psychologists have a number of options for treating depression, including anti-depressant medications, especially selective serotonin reuptake inhibitors, or SSRIs. But it's well known within psychiatry that as many as 66 percent of people with depression will not respond to the first medication they are prescribed.* In fact, patients are usually counseled early and often that their treatment might not work, and they might have to adjust their meds or switch types. This isn't to mention that this classification of medicines is notorious for significant side effects, as well as needing substantial time (sometimes upwards of four to eight weeks) to even assess if the proper dose of the proper medicine is working!

So how can it be that an SSRI that works for you might not work for me? The answer is simple: because we're different. My body chemistry reacts in a different way from yours. This is because of our genetics and because we all make different lifestyle choices and live in different environments and geographies, all of which can and do affect how our bodies handle medications, vitamins, surgeries, and everything else!

If this is true for SSRIs, isn't it true for everything we put into our bodies or every action we take? Of course, it is. But that's not how medicine tends to treat patients or is taught in medical schools. For an example, look at the treatment protocols for most major diseases: "If the patient has cholesterol levels above level X, then prescribe drug Y at Z dosage." This kind of "flowchart medicine" assumes that all patients will react the same way, even when we know that's not true.

And yet, for many reasons—lack of time, pervasive drug marketing, financial pressures—this is exactly the approach that most traditional doctors take (along with their physicians' associates, and nurse practitioners,

---

* WebMD. Treatment-resistant depression. https://www.webmd.com/depression/guide/treatment
  -resistant-depression-what-is-treatment-resistant-depression#1.

who may be doing the majority of patient care anyway). You're familiar with the expression, "If you're a hammer, then everything looks like a nail"? Too often, traditionally trained physicians are the hammer, and their patients are the nail—and thanks to rigidly enforced patient quotas, doctors know exactly how many nails they need to hit each day.

If this is true for pharmaceuticals, it's doubly true for so-called "alternative therapies." Why? Because of the way clinical trials and drug approval are set up in this country. Modern drug discovery wouldn't even be recognizable to Alexander Fleming and his petri dish of penicillin mold. Today, drug discovery is a highly sophisticated research operation conducted in the billion-dollar labs of a handful of pharmaceutical companies and richly funded biotech companies. A 2020 study in the *Journal of the American Medical Association (JAMA) Network* found that it cost between $985 million and $2.7 billion to bring a new drug to market. To arrive at this figure, researchers looked at all 355 new drugs and biologic agents approved by the Food and Drug Administration between 2009 and 2018.* The bulk of this cost is spent in drug discovery and the extensive clinical trials necessary to prove a drug has efficacy in humans and an acceptable safety profile.

By contrast, there is no billion-dollar industry working to prove that alternative therapies have efficacy. There are no billion-dollar marketing campaigns pushing people toward asking their doctors for alternative treatments. And perhaps most importantly, there is no money from alternative medicine companies flowing into our nation's medical schools. While this issue has gained little traction with the public, medical ethicists have spent at least the last two decades raising urgent warnings about the warping influence of pharmaceutical money on "academic medicine," meaning the universities and institutions where doctors are trained and therapies are studied.

One of the first shots in this skirmish between the public interest and the pharma/medical school industrial complex was memorably fired in 2000, when Marcia Angell, then editor of the prestigious *New England Journal of Medicine*, published an essay called "Is Academic Medicine for Sale?" Later a professor and lecturer at Harvard Medical School, Angell described the thorough corruption of the drug discovery process (more on this later) and medical education. Almost ten years after her essay—which landed her an interview with *60 Minutes*—Angell noted in a lecture at Harvard that a staggering 94 percent of physicians she surveyed have

* Wouters OJ, McKee M, Luyten J. Estimated research and development investment needed to bring a new medicine to market, 2009-2018. *JAMA*. 2020;323(9):844-853. doi:10.1001/jama.2020.1166.

reported taking direct money from the pharmaceutical industry, and that pharmaceutical companies were now designing their own drug discovery trials, including the ones that were ostensibly run by independent research groups at universities.*

Just one such example of how this works in real life occurred in 2006, when a report appeared in the *New England Journal of Medicine* describing a trial of three diabetes drugs and found that a drug called Avandia was the clear best option. Avandia was produced by pharmaceutical giant GlaxoSmithKline (2019 revenue: $43 billion), which promptly issued a statement saying its drug was "more effective" thanks to this "clear evidence." But it turned out the evidence wasn't so clear. The entire study that produced these results had been funded by GlaxoSmithKline, and every single one of the studies' eleven authors (all prestigious researchers) had received payments from Glaxo. Four of them were actually employed by the company and held stock. Perhaps not surprisingly, it turned out that this group of financially compromised researchers had produced a seriously flawed study, ignoring evidence that Avandia also increased the risk of heart attacks. Ultimately, a later study funded by the FDA showed that prescriptions of Avandia may have contributed to eighty-three thousand heart attacks and deaths, and the drug essentially vanished from the U.S. market.†

Far from being the exception, this kind of incestuous relationship between research institutions and medical research and education is the norm. Our recent history is littered with stories of drugs that should never have been approved but benefited from the paid-for loyalty of high-ranking academic researchers.

Stand back and let the full picture come into focus. Our medical schools are producing generations of doctors with hundreds of thousands of dollars in debt. They are attending medical schools that have been compromised by the influence of a flood of pharmaceutical money, which like all big money acts in its own self-interest without fail and ensures that medical education remains intensely focused on pharmaceuticals at the expense of so-called alternative therapies that lack deep-pocketed advocates.

The result? Generations of doctors that are ignorant (and skeptical) about the potential benefits of so-called alternative medicine and who have been

---

* Edmond J. Safra Center for Ethics, Harvard University. Drug companies and medicine: what money can buy. https://ethics.harvard.edu/event/drug-companies-and-medicine-what-money-can-buy.8
† Washington Post. (2012, November 12). As drug industry's influence over research grows, so does the potential for bias. https://www.washingtonpost.com/business/economy/as-drug-industrys-influence-over-research-grows-so-does-the-potential-for-bias/2012/11/24/bb64d596-1264-11e2-be82-c3411b7680a9_story.html.

Duke Makes Baby Steps

There's no doubt medical education in the United States has been hostile to alternative therapies, and we have a long way to go to correct that. But despite the grim situation, there are some indications it's changing at forward-thinking schools. One such example is the Duke Integrative Center in Raleigh Durham, North Carolina. This center has developed a medical training program that combines conventional and alternative therapies. The mission is defined as emphasizing prevention and wellness and promoting treatments that "address the whole person—mind, body, spirit, and community."*

---

* https://dukeintegrativemedicine.org/programs-training/public/for-those-who -hurt/.

---

trained to reach for the prescription pad at the first complaint without taking the time to fully assess patients and understand their medical etiologies.

This alarming gap in medical education has been well documented. In 2019, one of the world's leading medical journals, *The Lancet*, released a comprehensive study on the quality of nutrition education in medical schools. Researchers first noted "the centrality of nutrition to healthy lifestyle," then scoured the literature and medical school curriculum at various schools for evidence that medical students were learning about this critical area. Not surprisingly, they found that almost no medical schools provided "high-quality, effective nutrition care" and went on to recommend that medical schools need to provide "institutional support" for this area.* And keep in mind, this is education on something as basic as nutrition, which would include healthy diet alongside nutraceuticals and supplementation. When it comes to staying healthy, this is pretty basic stuff.

If something as basic as nutrition is not being discussed in our medical schools, then more advanced alternative approaches to managing health are also not being discussed. If we can't get our medical school programs to talk about something simple like nutrition, how can we get them to open their minds to other functional and regenerative medicine principles. The simple answer is we can't unless we change the schools themselves.

From a medical school's point of view, this makes sense—if you consider that modern medical education is the product of entrenched interests that all have a critical financial interest in what these young doctors will be

---

* Crowley J, Ball L, Hiddink GJ. Nutrition in medical education: a systematic review. Lancet Planet Health. 2019;3(9):e379-e389.

saying and prescribing when they get out of school. The simple truth is that teaching patients to proactively take control of their own health and learn to prevent disease and manage chronic conditions with low-impact therapies doesn't make much money. In other words, no matter what individual doctors may say, the larger medical industry doesn't want fully autonomous, empowered patients.

At the same time, individual doctors emerge from medical school seriously disadvantaged when it comes to any sort of alternative health practices. Learning to use alternative modalities in a clinical setting requires re-learning how medicine should work and partially undoing that $200,000 education the doctor is probably still paying off and has been "brainwashed" to follow. It means learning how these therapies really work, which means a thorough grounding in understanding how nutraceuticals interact with the body and with different disease states, how alternative modalities like bioidentical hormone optimization therapy and functional medicine operate, and most importantly, how all of these things can work together. In short, it means re-learning everything that was taught in medical school to be more focused on the whole patient and more accepting of whole-health treatments that not only attack individual diseases, but correct underlying problems like systemic inflammation or immune-system dysfunction that contribute to these conditions.

Naturally, most practitioners never make the effort to unwind the bad training they received in medical school, resulting in stubborn opposition to therapies that can make a huge difference in their patients' lives. And they'll have the full support of their medical institution, which is likely dictating how many patients they see every day and what treatment protocols they need to use. There is no way under these circumstances to spend real time with patients to understand what their unique biology, history, and lifestyle are like, along with gaining a deep understanding of how conditions that may seem disparate, like autoimmune GI conditions and coronary artery disease, are fundamentally connected by underlying disease factors that can be measured, treated, and tracked.

Unfortunately, there is very little national momentum in our current climate to rethink the many ways medical education stacks that deck against both doctors and patients. The cost of medical school is expected to keep rising, and the pervasive and rotting influence of the pharmaceutical industry will only grow as industry lobbying continues unchecked. Instead, it will be up to individuals to regain their autonomy, both doctors and patients. Physicians have an individual responsibility to learn about the many ways disease can be treated beyond the prescription pad and create practices that are truly focused on the patient.

Mostly, however, it's once again up to patients to take control of their own futures and seek out those enterprising healthcare providers who do understand how to unite traditional allopathic medicine and alternative medicine and create customized, personal health and wellness programs for their patients. This is a lot to ask from patients, but there's ample evidence that patients want to be treated with dignity, learn more about less-intensive therapies that not only treat their symptoms but connect with their whole health, and work with healthcare providers who can help them create individualized health plans. Ultimately, we live in a capitalist society, which means that voting with dollars is the most effective way to force change on a moribund medical industry. When enough patients and practitioners finally are willing to say, "ENOUGH!" then perhaps finally we will begin to design the healthcare system Americans deserve.

Chapter 3

Too Many Specialists, Not Enough Communication

"The body is one integrated system, not a collection of organs divided up by medical specialties. The medicine of the future connects everything."

—Mark Hyman, M.D.

Right now in the United States, there are roughly between 1 million and 1.2 million doctors practicing medicine, including specialists and doctors who received education overseas but are board certified to treat in the United States.* Although this is a five-fold increase from 1950, most experts agree this isn't enough doctors to keep America healthy and that we're headed for a demographic time bomb as the population continues to age and there aren't enough doctors to treat an older and sicker population.

---

* Statista. Total number of doctors of medicine in the U.S. from 1949 to 2015. https://www.statista.com/statistics/186260/total-doctors-of-medicine-in-the-us-since-1949/.

But even this obscures an underlying and more troublesome worry. Of those practicing doctors, just over half are specialists, meaning they have obtained additional education and are board-certified in a specialty such as orthopedics, cardiology, oncology, or anesthesiology. The rest are so-called generalists, including family doctors, general practitioners and internists, geriatricians, and general pediatricians.* If you remove the fifty-eight thousand pediatricians,† who are obviously narrowly focused on children, this widens the gap a bit more, resulting in a lopsided count between specialists and general physicians.

With this in mind, consider that most Americans receive their general medical care from one of two sources: either the emergency room or via general practitioners. The evolution of general medical care into the emergency room is itself a major problem—every year, about 20 percent of American adults visit an emergency room, resulting in 141 million emergency department visits. This represents a 34 percent increase in emergency room visits between 1995 and 2019, which is roughly double the rate we'd expect to see based on population growth.‡

Under these dry statistics is a pressing question: why are so many adults relying on the emergency room for routine, non-emergency medical visits? The answer may lie in the second way Americans seek out routine medical care, through general practitioners. The fact is, there aren't enough general practitioners in the United States to keep up with an aging population that is suffering from an explosion of chronic diseases, especially those related to burgeoning obesity rates. The general practitioners who are still working are so overcrowded that it can take ninety days to see the doctor, which is what motivates patients to go to the emergency room. The Association of American Medical Colleges estimates that the United States will have a shortage of between twenty-one thousand and fifty-five thousand primary care physicians by 2032.§

This shortage plays out in a real way for millions of American patients every year. If you've ever switched insurance plans (and who hasn't in

---

* Statista. Number of active physicians in the U.S. 2020 by specialty area. https://www.statista.com/statistics/209424/us-number-of-active-physicians-by-specialty-area/.
† American Academy of Pediatrics. What is a Pediatrician? https://www.aap.org/en-us/professional-resources/Pediatrics-as-a-Profession/Pages/Frequently-Asked-Questions.aspx.
‡ Becker's Hospital Review. Emergency department overuse: routing low-acuity visits away from the ED with virtual care. https://www.beckershospitalreview.com/healthcare-information-technology/emergency-department-overuse-routing-low-acuity-visits-away-from-the-ed-with-virtual-care.html.
§ Washington Post. (2019, July 15). America to face a shortage of primary care physicians within a decade or so. https://www.washingtonpost.com/health/america-to-face-a-shortage-of-primary-care-physicians-within-a-decade-or-so/2019/07/12/0cf144d0-a27d-11e9-bd56-eac6bb02d01d_story.html.

recent years, considering the chaos in the insurance markets?), or moved to a new city, you're no doubt familiar with the challenge of finding a new general practitioner. It's not uncommon for people in a new plan to receive a list of participating general internists or family doctors, only to find that none of these offices are currently accepting patients, or there is a ten- to twelve-week wait for a new patient appointment. It's no wonder more and more Americans are turning to the emergency department or using the walk-in clinics that seem to be springing up in every convenience store, strip mall, or big-box retailer around the country.

Unfortunately, this movement away from a "family doctor" has dire health consequences, especially when it's considered in light of the truly shocking chaos that is our country's medical record system. A patient who goes into a walk-in clinic or an ED for a complaint has no reasonable expectation that the results of this visit will be added to any medical record to be considered in the course of future treatment. Instead, if the patient wants to make sure he or she actually has a comprehensive medical record, they'll have to track down their own medical records after the incident is over and physically carry these documents into their future doctors' visits.

The result is a near total lack of continuity in care where patients are plunged into a system of such mind-boggling complexity that even insiders have trouble making sense out of it and the idea of whole-person care that evolves with an individual is laughable. Especially for patients with multiple diagnoses, there is almost no chance their medical information will follow them through the system, so every new doctor has to rely on the patient for accurate reporting or basically start over. If practitioners were consistent about tracking down medical records, that would be helpful— but for the most part, doctors rarely take the effort to find their patient's complete medical history and actually communicate with other doctors who have seen the same patient, nor do they have the time to chase records down and review a complex individual's records.

This is bad enough, but to really understand the complexity and its incredible cost, we have to next look at the other side of the equation. As I noted in the opening of this chapter, a little under half of all physicians in the United States are generalists, meaning that over half of all practicing doctors are specialists. Overall, this means there are just over 535,000 specialists practicing in the United States.*

---

* Statista. Number of active physicians in the U.S. 2020 by specialty area. https://www.statista.com/ statistics/209424/us-number-of-active-physicians-by-specialty-area/.

For defenders of the status quo, this is something worth bragging about. When people say, "The United States has the best medical care in the world," what they actually mean is that the United States has the most specialists, and some of the most advanced specialists in the world. It makes a great soundbite, but unfortunately this glib statement actually masks one of the most pressing problems in medicine today: we are way too focused on specialists.

This heavy emphasis on specialists makes sense for individual physicians, who are pushed toward specialties from their earliest days in medical schools and know that specialists often get paid higher amounts of money, which sounds attractive to a broke college student. As it turns out, most of the top-rated medical schools are associated with academic centers like universities and university hospitals. The focus of these institutions is firmly placed on producing more specialists, not least because that's the best way to increase the amount of revenue a medical school can squeeze from every student. Remember how the average medical school costs about $140,000 for a four-year degree, not counting expenses like books, housing, and food? At the end of this process, medical students will get their MD, but for many that's only the beginning of the process. Becoming a specialist will require landing an internal medicine residency, during which time the young doctor will go through multiple clinical rotations while working under conditions that are often described as barbaric. It's not uncommon to hear doctors talking about their residencies in terms usually reserved for combat soldiers, sometimes with the same swagger.

And why not? Up until 2003, there was no limit to how many hours residents could work. This situation began to change when the cost of treating residents like slaves started to become apparent. Residents routinely were working twenty-four- or thirty-six-hours shifts. Naturally, this wasn't good for either residents or their patients. In 1999, a study found that as many as ninety thousand people died every year thanks to preventable medical errors, and resident work hours were singled out as a major cause of these errors.* When news of this finally reached the public, the United States government was prodded into action. In 2003, Congress passed laws that capped the number of hours a resident could work to a still-astounding eighty hours per week, with shifts capped at thirty hours. The reward for this work? In 2019, residents earned an average of $61,200 annually.†

* Kevin MD. The evolution of resident work hours. https://www.kevinmd.com/blog/2018/11/the-evolution-of-residents-hours.html.

† Medscape. Medscape residents salary & debt report 2019. https://www.medscape.com/slideshow/2019-residents-salary-debt-report-6011735.

Modern residency has a coming-of-age or rite-of-passage feel as well, which ensures this ridiculous practice will never change. Residents must report to an attending supervising physician, who typically has a very "authoritative" teaching style. Later, as that resident advances and goes out into the world to become an attending physician themselves, they will feel the need to carry on this approach with their residents, and the problem is never corrected.

Meanwhile, residencies typically last three years, although they can last up to seven years for more complex specialties. And that's not the end of the line for specialists. After completing a residency, many specialties require fellowships. Unlike a residency, which is a more general exposure to medical practice, the fellowship is a tightly focused program in the doctor's preferred specialty. Fellowships typically last another three years, depending on the specialty. During a fellowship, the fellow will be intensively trained in their chosen specialty. At this point, the working conditions may improve somewhat—the candidate will probably not be working eighty-hour weeks any longer—but the pay is still low. Depending on their specialty, fellows typically earn between $51,000 and about $75,000 a year.*

And even this may not be the end. For physicians who are interested in obtaining a sub-specialty, there may be another year or more of training before they can earn board certification in their desired specialty.

By the time the physician is done with all of this training, they have been in school or training programs for ten years or more, often experiencing grueling working conditions. So why would anyone go through this? Perhaps it's the dream of their specialty bringing them goodwill and fortune? It must, in order to overcome everything they just endured, right?

Here's where the real problems with this system start to emerge. Not surprisingly, the act of specializing is exactly that: a narrowing of focus. A popular joke among doctors goes like this: "The same patient goes to a surgeon, a cryo-ablationist, and an endocrinologist and is surprised to find out they need surgery, ablation, and hormone treatments." Why would this be? Because after spending ten years focused only on one narrow avenue for treatment, why would a physician recommend anything else? Like I said earlier, to a hammer, everything looks like a nail. To a doctor who has been steeped in one narrow specialty, everything looks like that condition. Similarly, if you were to ask ten different doctors their opinion on the same patient, chances are you would get ten different answers! Thanks

---

* The Atlantic. (2015, January 27). What doctors make. https://www.theatlantic.com/health/archive/2015/01/physician-salaries/384846/.

to specialization, doctors' minds are often "warped" into tying patients' medical conditions into their specialty so they can "do something" for the patient, even if it's not the optimal approach!

And from here it only gets worse. Remember the earlier example of patients who use walk-in clinics or the ER for primary care, but don't have a comprehensive medical record or continuity of care? This problem is much, much worse among the specialties, especially for patients with complex care conditions, which is most of them. No matter how the system is set up—with doctors pursuing a laser focus on their own specialty or condition—it doesn't change the way people age and get sick. The truth is that disease rarely happens in a vacuum; when people fall victim to a chronic disease, it usually doesn't happen in isolation. Consider:

- 40 percent of patients with heart failure also have diabetes.*

- More than 50 percent of patients with chronic kidney disease have hypertension.†

- 25 percent of people with cancer develop a major depressive disorder.‡

- 75 percent of patients with non-alcoholic fatty liver disease have diabetes.

The list could go on almost endlessly, but the point is simple: chronic, serious diseases rarely happen in a vacuum. In the real world—not the cloistered world of modern medical training—chronic diseases are often the product of complex processes and conditions that affect the whole body and many organ systems, leading to a more generalized breakdown in cellular processes and tissue health that finally manifests in one or more disease. And because these specialists are so narrow-minded, they fail to recognize the global contributing factors to the disease process that may be coming from an organ system outside of the specialist's organ system! This is compounded by the fact that specialists often lose a lot of their

---

* Seferović PM, Petrie MC, Filippatos GS, et al. Type 2 diabetes mellitus and heart failure: a position statement from the Heart Failure Association of the European Society of Cardiology. *Eur J Heart Fail.* 2018;20(5):853-872.

† National Kidney Foundation. High blood pressure and chronic kidney disease. https://www.kidney.org/sites/default/files/docs/hbpandckd.pdf.

‡ American Cancer Society. Depression. https://www.cancer.org/treatment/treatments-and-side-effects/physical-side-effects/emotional-mood-changes/depression.html.

generalized medical knowledge and insight, thanks to years of intense focus. Specialists don't often feel obligated or responsible to help manage general health concerns. And with so many patients skipping general practitioners, how can they possibly get better when their doctors (specialists) are only focused on one organ system? Specialists take the same Hippocratic oath as any practitioner, yet they are often the first to dismiss or ignore the patient's underlying health issues if it falls outside of the specialist's scope of practice. In fact, specialists are often notoriously known for encouraging patients to "follow up with your primary for that." This is especially true when being seen in an ER or walk-in clinic. Keeping in mind, most of the time the patient is in the ER or walk-in clinic is because they *cannot* be seen by their primary. Not to mention, as we've discussed, not only is there a shortage of primary care practitioners, there are also insurance and network rules and guidelines to follow, and sometimes ninety-day wait times to see your primary, all because these specialists are ignoring the same Hippocratic oath that all healthcare practitioners take, which is to help our patients in any way possible.

Continuity of Care: The Missing Ingredient

This problem is made much worse by the lack of continuity of care. Specialists not only frequently fail to track down a patient's medical record, but they also rarely communicate with each other even on the same case. The lack of communication is a very, very big problem as patients are misdiagnosed, under-treated, or prescribed medications that can react with one another (to name a few smaller issues).

Even among the specialists who are interested in better communication, there are structural obstacles to communication between various specialists. These include patient privacy concerns like HIPAA, which was created to give patients more control over their own medical information, but also from commercial concerns from the entities that control medical information. Not surprisingly, managing medical information is a huge business in the United States, and the companies that build the platforms hospitals use to track patient information through electronic medical records (EMRs) are fiercely resistant to opening their systems up and making it easier for different specialties to communicate with each other. It took a federal mandate to force companies like Epic and Cerner, which control the vast majority of the hospital-based EMR business in the United

States, to open their platforms—and even then, they are erecting obstacles to transparency that is slowing the easy flow of medical information through the system. And this isn't even to mention that none of these EMR systems communicate with each other, even among single hospitals that use multiple EMRs!

So how does this affect individual patients? Imagine this common example: let's say Bob, a fifty-one-year-old, goes into his general practitioner and complains about "feeling down." In the office, he's given a screening evaluation for depression, and there's enough concern that his doctor refers him to a psychiatrist. Bob finds a psychiatrist that takes his insurance and goes in for evaluation (after being forced to wait sixty days). The psychiatrist finds that Bob is indeed suffering from symptoms consistent with major depression and prescribes a selective-serotonin reuptake inhibitor (SSRI).

Unfortunately, however, Bob is among the majority of patients for whom their first prescriptions don't work, and not only does his depression deepen, he starts to experience side effects like sleeplessness, irritability, and weight gain. He tells his psychiatrist what's going on, and the psychiatrist writes a referral for an endocrinologist to evaluate Bob's blood sugars and hormone status. This likely should have been the first step, but again, specialists usually stick to their lane, which in this case means a prescription for depression. At the endocrinologist, Bob is given a standard hormone test, where he's found to be "normal" for his age for testosterone and other sex hormones. The endocrinologist tells Bob it's not his hormones after all and sends him back to the psychiatrist, who concludes that Bob needs a drug that aids in mood stability and prescribes a second type of antidepressant with its own side effects that contributes to the side effects from the original SSRI.

This second SSRI doesn't work either, and Bob steadily becomes more depressed assuming his depression can't be treated. Bob then goes back to his GP, who runs a new set of blood tests and discovers that Bob's cholesterol and liver function tests are abnormal. The GP refers Bob to a gastroenterologist to evaluate these new liver and cholesterol abnormalities, which are likely due to the two SSRI antidepressants Bob is taking, but because no one is communicating on Bob's behalf, this gets missed. The GI specialist runs a slew of tests, exposing Bob to radiation, contrast, and adding more drugs to his regimen. Unfortunately, none of this helps, and Bob now is feeling worse and worse. In fact, now he's concerned about even bigger problems. The GI doctor was concerned about "a benign incidental finding" on one of his diagnostic tests and is talking about cancer or surgery....

You can see how this goes on and on. In all of this back and forth, not one of Bob's doctors shares records with the others. Bob's original general practitioner has to rely on Bob himself to find out what's going on, and because Bob is on his company's insurance, he's worried about sharing a diagnosis of depression with a GP in case it might get back to his employer. And of course, the psychiatrist and endocrinologist only "communicate" with each other through Bob himself in a game of a telephone tag where the middleman (Bob) has no medical education and only a rudimentary understanding of how depression, hormones, and prescription drugs all work together, but he has no choice but to accept and go along with what his specialists are telling him.

At the end of the day, Bob has no continuity of care. He's treated individually by multiple practitioners who never bother to learn or even simply speak with each other. Naturally, his treatment fails, and he's lost months pursuing treatment through multiple appointments, spent several hundred or thousand dollars, and, worst of all, blames himself for failing to respond to treatment and sinks deeper into depression.

This kind of thing happens every day, thousands of times across the United States. Patients are hustled through a system that looks at the most obvious symptoms and responds with the most convenient pharmaceutical intervention or surgery available. Specialists operating in silos advocate for their specialty, and virtually no part of the system communicates with any other part. No one takes the time to connect the dots between disparate symptoms and address underlying causes. There is little or no continuity of care.

In Bob's case, it turns out that a relatively simple examination could have uncovered what was going on. It turns out that Bob's depression— which arose despite him seeming healthy and not experiencing any sort of trauma—was the manifestation of several underlying causes: inflammation and age-related changes to Bob's hormone levels. A rapidly emerging body of research is finding that immune-mediated inflammation can play a major role in depression and other mental health conditions, and even affect the body's natural hormone production and balance. It turns out that chronic inflammation and elevation of inflammatory blood factors changes the brain chemistry and makes patients vulnerable to clinical depression.* We now know that inflammation contributes to the degradation of male hormones and increases estrogen production, which tends to affect men cognitively.

---

* Lee CH, Giuliani F. The role of inflammation in depression and fatigue. *Front Immunol.* 2019;10:1696. Published 2019 Jul 19. doi:10.3389/fimmu.2019.01696.

In fact, Bob's "mental illness" could have been treated with an anti-inflammatory and hormone-balancing regimen that included nutraceuticals, hormone therapy, and other approaches that lack the side effects of SSRIs.

And it goes even deeper than that! Not only was underlying immune-system activation affecting Bob's mental health, his chronic inflammation was also damaging the arteries in his heart, raising his risk for atherosclerosis and a heart attack. Without some kind of comprehensive intervention, it's almost inevitable that Bob would someday soon end up in a cardiologist's office, where he would be prescribed another medication like a statin to "protect" his heart. This would leave Bob taking a handful of pills every day, still fighting his depression, feeling confused and adrift in a medical industry where no one seems to be communicating and no one can tell him what's "wrong" with him, and now watching the clock anxiously for a heart attack.

The sad truth is this type of thing is common, and millions of patients are struggling to navigate this system, even though its flaws are well known. The issue is that fixing it would require taking on some of the most entrenched and richest corporate and academic interests in the country. The fact that medical information is siloed is not a bug in the system—it's a feature. Billion-dollar corporations have an entrenched interest in ensuring they can build the software platforms that house this information and cut out competition. Healthcare networks have a vested interest in making sure patients don't go elsewhere for care. Privacy laws meant to protect patients have the effect of stifling the flow of information and throwing responsibility onto patients—setting them up to be unsuccessful because patients will not be able to navigate the system and will be forced to comply. And our entire medical education and training infrastructure is geared to produce as many specialists as possible, most of whom enter practice burdened with extraordinary debt and little training on the business aspects of medicine.

This last point must be emphasized once again: it's not fair to blame individual doctors who choose to pursue specialties for the weaknesses in this system. In fact, those doctors are trapped in the same system patients are stuck with, and they are making rational choices based on the economic reality of medicine today. The truth is, of the top-ten best-paying salaried jobs in the United States, eight of them are medical specialties. These include anesthesiologist, surgeons and oral surgeons, OB/GYNs, and psychiatrists.* For some sub-specialties, the average salaries are truly

---

* Business Insider. (2020, April 20). The 30 highest-paying jobs in America. https://www.businessinsider.com/highest-paying-jobs-in-america-2019-2#1-anesthesiologists-30.

eye-popping: an interventional cardiologist can expect to make an average of $343,000 annually once they start practicing.* When staring down the barrel of a six-figure student loan and a profession wracked with liability problems, it's only natural that doctors-in-training would aim for the highest-paying specialties in medicine.

Whatever the reason, though, the end result is the same: a system that is hopelessly complex and makes it nearly impossible for patients to experience comprehensive continuity of care, with care typically fragmented between specialists who have little or no communication, except through the patients themselves. Worse yet, it's a system that functions worse the sicker the patient is, because they'll need to see more specialists. The risk here for patients is real. It shows up in missed diagnoses, neglected underlying factors that are causing or contributing to disease, and overlapping prescriptions that increase the chances of a dangerous drug cross-reaction.

Ultimately, patients are on their own but not empowered. Rather than confidently charting their own course and proactively managing their own health, too many patients feel like they're drowning, unsure of what they can do to help their own care, nervous they'll end up incurring tens or even hundreds of thousands of dollars in medical debt, and drowning in the administrative complexity of navigating our healthcare system. Fixing this broken system is an urgent national priority on every level.

---

* Glassdoor. (2019, December 1). Interventional cardiologist salaries. https://www.glassdoor.com/Salaries/interventional-cardiologist-salary-SRCH_KO0,27.htm.

Chapter 4

Hospital Consolidation for Profits, not Patients

"Hospitals are self-fueling, ever-expanding machines. There is an infinite amount of stuff to buy — amenities, machines, new wings, higher salaries, more nurses. If you pay hospitals more, they spend it. If you pay them less, they adjust. The only way to pay less for healthcare is to pay less for healthcare."

—James Robinson

Watch enough old TV and at some point you'll see an idealized version of medical care from a bygone era. In those days, the doctor was invariably a kindly older gentleman with a black bag, who actually made house calls when someone was sick. If something was more serious, but not urgent, he'd recommend the patient come into his office for a more thorough examination. The "office" was usually a small practice or even a solo practice with the doctor's name on the letterhead and the door. If things were really serious, the patient might be taken to a hospital, where the same doctor had treating privileges and would visit there to continue care. The doctor also knew about you, your family, and had formed an actual relationship with you.

This version of our medical system is embedded deep in our cultural memory—but it bears little resemblance to the way medicine operates in today's world. The reality is that medicine is the biggest business in the United States, and like any large business, there is incredible pressure on the system to create administrative efficiencies and competitive advantages with a focus on delivering consistent profits to the shareholders and investors.

This shows up most obviously in hospital consolidation—an area that few people outside the industry pay attention to but has boomed over the last 20 years as huge health networks gobble up smaller and nonprofit hospitals. In 2019, there were 768 mergers and acquisitions across the healthcare industry, an almost 10 percent increase from the year before. These transactions fell into a few categories, including:

- Large systems buying "distressed hospitals" with the object of cutting costs and streamlining operations to restore profitability.

- Investments in healthcare technology, including major plays by consumer-focused technology companies like Amazon and Apple to shoulder into the lucrative healthcare business.

- Thanks to changes in the way Medicare reimburses long-term care (LTC) and home health, there was a surge in mergers among home health companies "away from the mom-and-pop entities" (read: smaller, more personal businesses) that were once common.

- Continued consolidation among the diagnostic and lab companies that process the majority of the nation's blood tests and other diagnostic tests.*

Among these mergers was the so-called "mega-merger" between healthcare giants CVS and Aetna. In late 2019, the U.S. government approved CVS Health Corp.'s $70 billion acquisition of health insurance giant Aetna Inc. At first glance, this might seem like a strange pairing: why would a drugstore operator like CVS have any interest in getting into the insurance business? And why was the merger greeted with alarm among antitrust activists and government agencies, who promptly raised concerns of "vertical

---

* Hammond Hanlon Camp, LLC. (2020, January 28). "H2C industry insights: 2019 in review. https:// www.h2c.com/2019-in-review-healthcare-ma.

monopolies"? Why did news of this merger prompt American Medical Association (AMA) President Patrice Harris, MD, to write, "It's hard to find any upside to a merger that leaves [patients] with fewer choices"?*

The answer, of course, has little to do with patient care and everything to do with economics. Simply put, CVS Health, already the largest pharmacy in the country (revenue: $109 billion), wanted to also own the insurance company that covers the medications its patients buy. This allows CVS/Aetna to reap greater profits by removing the middleman between the pharmacy and payor. Obviously, as Dr. Harris of the AMA pointed out, there's little chance any of these savings will be passed along to patients— and every chance in the world that Aetna will leverage its newfound power to pad its own bottom line.

Almost immediately after the merger, reports began to pop up online of consumers saying that Aetna was refusing to cover certain drugs , supplies, or procedures unless the patient went to CVS. Examples included refusing to pay for flu shots or other medications. In 2020, Aetna formalized this pressure campaign by announcing new plans to "nudge" patients toward CVS through a new plan called Aetna Connected. The development was alarming enough that David Balto, a former policy director with the Federal Trade Commission, remarked that, "CVS is moving toward a restricted market approach that would only be attractive to the Soviet Union."†

While few consumers pay close attention to this merger and acquisitions activity, it literally affects every American who uses the healthcare system and not just hospitals. What's happening with alarming speed is the rapid vertical consolidation of the medical industry into huge healthcare networks. These networks are spreading into every area where healthcare is delivered, providing end-to-end care for American patients, including physician practices, walk-in clinics, rehab facilities, and even home health.

The standard response from hospital and healthcare companies to criticism of this torrid pace of merger and acquisitions is that it's necessary to maintain a competitive advantage. After all, the United States enjoys a form of regulated capitalism that thrives on competition. According to this logic, survival depends on aggressive growth to stake out market share and defend against competitors, who themselves are also growing quickly through mergers and acquisitions. In other words, if you want to be a big fish, you have to eat a lot of little fish.

---

* Medical Economics. (2019, September 5). CVS-Aetna merger approved. https://www.medicaleconomics.com/view/coronavirus-feds-extend-public-health-emergency-declaration.

† HealthcareDive. Aetna unveils plan nudging members to CVS clinics, pharmacies. https://www.healthcaredive.com/news/aetna-unveils-plan-nudging-members-to-cvs-clinics-pharmacies/584475/.

This seems like it makes sense on the surface, and it's certainly true in other industries where size and customer reach are closely related. But there's another side to this argument that doesn't get nearly as much attention as it should, mostly because the people who are qualified to make it are underfunded and lack the multi-billion-dollar platform of a huge healthcare company. This counterargument is rooted in the simple principle that all of this competitive activity isn't really aimed at improving patient care but is instead squarely aimed at enriching big players in the healthcare industry itself.

If this counterargument is true, then it would follow that patient care hasn't really improved but profitability has. And guess what? That's exactly the scenario we're seeing unfolding now. As noted earlier, our health outcomes in the United States are actually going backward. Our life expectancy in this country is dropping, despite the fact that we're the richest country on earth with the most technologically advanced healthcare sector. As also noted, medical bills are the leading cause of bankruptcy. And our overall health outcomes border on shameful. In 2015, the Commonwealth Fund did a deep analysis comparing the United States healthcare system to eleven industrialized, high-income countries, including Australia, Canada, France, German, the Netherlands, New Zealand, Norway, Sweden, Switzerland, and the United Kingdom. Here's what they found:

- We spend nearly twice as much per capita on healthcare as these countries yet have the lowest life expectancy and the highest suicide rate.

- We have the highest disease burden from chronic diseases, with an obesity rate that's almost twice the average.

- Americans are much less likely to visit the physician than people in other countries, in part because of the inability to pay for it or fear of high medical bills.

- Once a patient does go to the doctor, they are much more likely to be referred for an expensive diagnostic test.

- The United States suffers from the highest number of hospitalizations from preventable causes and the highest rate of avoidable deaths.*

---

* Commonwealth Fund. (2020, January 30). U.S. health care from a global perspective, 2019: higher spending, worse outcomes? https://www.commonwealthfund.org/publications/issue-briefs/2020/jan/us-health-care-global-perspective-2019.

This depressing picture hardly supports the idea that we're "getting the most for our money" from our healthcare system. So, if patients aren't seeing the benefits of all those billions spent, who is? After all, it's well documented that healthcare expenses are rising much faster than inflation or wages. Certainly, that money is going somewhere.

Indeed, it is. It will come as no surprise to find out that, by any measure, healthcare is one of the most profitable sectors in the entire U.S. economy. Almost every sector of the U.S. healthcare industry has been enjoying huge profits year after year for the last several years. Here are just a few results:

- In 2019, the insurance industry enjoyed an increasing gap between revenue from premiums versus the increase in benefits, resulting in soaring profits of $913 billion for the seven largest publicly traded health insurance companies.*

- Nowhere are profits higher than the pharmaceutical industry, where it's not uncommon for drug makers to reap profits of 20 percent on total revenue.†

While it's true that hospitals tend to operate on tighter profit margins, often in the single digits, it still matters where these profits go. And guess what? It turns out that most of them go into investors' pockets or, increasingly, into the pockets of senior executives. A 2018 study found that CEOs and CFOs of healthcare companies enjoyed pay increases of more than 90 percent over a ten-year period from 2008 to 2018.‡ For larger systems, this translates into eye-popping annual salary packages. In 2019, the CEO of Hospital Corporation of America, Samuel N. Hazen, earned a cool $26.7 million. If there's a bright side to this frankly outrageous compensation, perhaps it's that it will motivate pharmaceutical giant Merck's CEO, Kenneth Frazier, to work harder, considering he only made $22.5 million in 2019.

It's worth stopping here to let these numbers really soak in. Considering the poor state of healthcare in this country—we've already seen we spend more and get worse outcomes—is there really any justification for one

---

* Benefits Pro, (2020, February 24, 2020). Top health insurer's revenues soared to almost $1 trillion in 2019. https://www.benefitspro.com/2020/02/24/top-health-insurers-revenues-soared-to-almost -1-trillion-in-2019/?slreturn=20200626180107.

† U.S. Government Accountability Office. Drug industry. https://www.gao.gov/products/GAO-18-40.

‡ Healthcare Finance. (2020, January 16). Study sheds light on executive pay in the healthcare industry. https://www.healthcarefinancenews.com/news/study-sheds-light-executive-pay-healthcare-industry.

person to earn that much in a single year? No doubt Mr. Hazen and Mr. Frazier are good at their jobs, but are they really returning almost $50 million worth of value annually to America's patients? The obvious answer is no, because they weren't hired to return value to patients. They were hired to return value to shareholders, plain and simple. And what's the best way to do that? More mergers, more acquisitions, less competition, and providing the most expensive care at every juncture. It's a slow-moving tragedy that's inflicted on patients 24 hours a day, 365 days a year.

So far, we've examined the industry as a whole, but let's dig deeper and see what effects this is having on the delivery of healthcare at the physician and patient level. Here's where the real cost of this tragedy starts to come into focus. Remember in the beginning of the chapter, our hypothetical doctor who ran a solo or small partner practice and knew his or her patients by name, often seeing the same family of patients for years and years? This antiquated version of medical care has also been overtaken by acquisitions and economics.

In 1983, just over 75 percent of physicians owned their own practices, according to a study by the American Medical Association. Faced with high administrative and liability costs, however, a trend emerged of doctors abandoning their own practices and signing on as employees of large healthcare networks and hospitals. By 1994, the number of doctors that owned their own practices had declined to 57.7 percent, and it was still dropping. By 2012, it was down to 53.2 percent, and in 2018, for the first time in U.S. history, the number of doctors who owned their own practices fell below 50 percent, with only 47.4 percent of doctors having an ownership share in their practice.*

There's nothing inherently wrong with physicians making the choice to shutter a private practice and go to work for a hospital or healthcare network—but this is happening with little or no thought put to the consequences of the shift, and it's happening at such a rapid rate that there eventually will be no more solo or small practices. The data that is emerging about the effect this has on patient care, costs, and the physicians themselves is so far not encouraging.

According to research from the independent data company Geneia, doctors working in corporate or hospital-owned organizations are more

---

* MarketWatch. (2019, May 8). For the first time, physicians are less likely to operate their own practices. https://www.marketwatch.com/story/for-the-first-time-physicians-are-less-likely-to-operate-their-own-practices-2019-05-08.

likely to report burnout, cynicism with their jobs, reduced empathy toward their patients, and deviating from clinical guidelines in care delivery.*

Hospital-owned physician practices are much more likely to refer patients for expensive diagnostic testing, with some practices registering an astonishing 83 to 205 percent increase in referrals for diagnostic testing.† This raises the overall cost of healthcare for consumers, and there is significant debate in the medical community that over-testing is rampant throughout the system.

As hospitals consolidate with each other and buy up physician practices, the rise of "super-concentrated" markets with only one or two options for consumers makes it harder for new providers to enter the market, meaning power is consolidated and there is little pressure to lower prices.‡

As discouraging as this early data is, the fact is that we don't fully understand the effects this accelerating consolidation will have or is currently having. The trend toward consolidation is relatively new, and our healthcare system is so large and complex that it can be very difficult to track any outcome or change back to one single cause. Nevertheless, there are urgent and pressing questions that still need to be answered when it comes to this rapid vertical (hospitals buying physician practices) and horizontal (hospitals buying hospitals) consolidation among healthcare entities. These include its real-world effect on prices for consumers, physician satisfaction, competition, access to the market for new providers, quality of care, and patient satisfaction.

There is one area, however, where it's clear that consolidation and costs are having a profoundly dangerous and negative effect: rural healthcare. It's no exaggeration to say that rural healthcare is in full crisis in this country, a condition that has only be exacerbated by the coronavirus pandemic. Rural hospitals are uniquely vulnerable for many reasons. They tend to be smaller, without the kind of high-profit service lines that larger, metropolitan hospitals use to prop up their bottom lines, especially orthopedic and cardiac surgery units. Their patient population is often typically older with a greater chronic disease burden. At the same time, they are more likely to see a higher percentage of patients on Medicaid or Medicare, which typically pay

* Geneia. Employed physicians more dissastisfied than independent doctors.https://content.geneia.com/2018/independentdocshappier/index.html.

† Modern Healthcare. (2018, March 16). Rapid rise in hospital-employed physicians increases costs. https://www.modernhealthcare.com/article/20180316/TRANSFORMATION02/180319913/rapid-rise-in-hospital-employed-physicians-increases-costs.

‡ Healthcare Dive. (2019, November 7). Hospital M&A spurs rising healthcare costs, MedPAC finds. https://www.healthcaredive.com/news/hospital-ma-spurs-rising-healthcare-costs-medpac-finds/566858/.

lower reimbursement rates than private insurance. Finally, struggling rural hospitals have a much harder time attracting new physicians.

Due to a lack of access to care, rural hospitals often turn into a general practitioner's office as people flood the hospital for less acute concerns, which increases the burden on practitioners working in these environments. Instead of thinking about the long-term care of patients, overworked practitioners have to be in triage mode, with no time to focus on prevention, hence the patient never has the ability to get better and ends up repeating the same cycle of using the ER for acute exacerbations of chronic issues and receiving care from emergency doctors who are more concerned with stabilizing them than treating the underlying condition.

In a normal market, this situation would represent a market opportunity for new providers to move into a market and offer lower-cost alternatives. But that's not happening in rural America.

When a rural hospital closes, it can have immediate and serious health consequences for people living within in its service area—and rural hospitals are closing by the dozens. According to the American Academy of Family Physicians (AAFP), there have been more than a hundred rural hospital closures over the last ten years alone, with another several hundred that are teetering on the edge of bankruptcy. The result, says the AAFP, is the creation of "medical and obstetric deserts where there is no medical care for hundreds of miles. Most of these have been in communities with largely minority populations."* And we wonder why this country is so sick? These consolidation tactics make our country sicker as people lose access to quality care.

The real-world consequences of this includes increased infant mortality in rural areas, a lack of mental health and addiction treatment options in communities that are more likely to be ravaged by the opiate epidemic, and a dramatically increased risk of dying for poor minorities in rural areas. This is especially true for Native Americans, who have some of the worst health outcomes in the United States.†

There is no easy solution for this problem with many patients, but there's no doubt that this crisis is the leading edge and most visible outcome

---

* American Academy of Family Physicians. (2019, July 9). NEW AAFP initiative addresses rural health care crisis. https://www.aafp.org/news/blogs/leadervoices/entry/20190709lv-ruralhealth-matters.html.

† American Academy of Family Physicians. (2019, July 9). NEW AAFP initiative Addresses Rural Health Care Crisis. https://www.aafp.org/news/blogs/leadervoices/entry/20190709lv-ruralhealth-matters.html.

of all of the trends we've looked at so far, including consolidation and the lack of family physicians and generalists.

If the goal of a functioning medical system is to empower patients to take control of their own health and to provide them with the tools and knowledge needed to make good healthcare decisions in conjunction with their doctors, our country is failing miserably. In real ways, the deck is actually stacked against individual patients, who should be forgiven for being confused and overmatched by the trillion-dollar interests that have conspired against them. Truly, what can one patient do about a system that is designed to prioritize profits over patients? A system that has at its disposal tens of millions of dollars to feed into Washington and head off any meaningful anti-trust regulation?

While the government has made halting steps to protect patients' interests—like passing laws that make it somewhat harder for hospitals to snap up physician practices—ordinary patients lack the type of deep-pocketed, influential advocates that would be required to reshape our current system in a way that hands power and priority back to the people who need it most: you and me, us, the patients.

Chapter 5

Insurance: Denies by Design

"You can't afford to get sick, and you can't depend on the present health care system to keep you well."

—Dr. Andrew Weil

Ask most Americans what they think of the private insurance industry, and you're likely to hear an avalanche of complaints. The industry's image is so bad that even the industry has caught on—insurance trade magazines and publications are full of articles on how the industry can repair its image problem. In one recent example of this genre, the industry was described as looking "boring, stiff, greedy, and exclusive" in a column in a decidedly industry-friendly magazine.*

On a more academic note, the polling company YouGov recently studied perceptions of the insurance industry and found some interesting things:

- Just 50 percent of adults "respect" insurance companies.

- 72 percent of adults think the industry uses deliberately confusing language.

---

* Insurance Nerds. The insurance industry has an image problem. https://insnerds.com/image-problem/.

- Almost half of adults don't think the industry acts in patients' best interests, versus the 42 percent who think it does (the rest are undecided).*

These are damning numbers for an industry that's literally designed to provide health protection for people—but they shouldn't be surprising. Unfortunately, there are good reasons for the collapse in public confidence. The American healthcare system is unique among advanced nations for several reasons, most notably the fact that the majority of people get private insurance through their employer, instead of relying on a national healthcare system. The effect is that health insurance is tied to employment, and employers are understandably anxious to reduce this major cost center whenever they can.

There are historical reasons for this that are beyond the scope of this book, but the end result is that our insurance system is fundamentally broken, even if insurance companies themselves remain financially healthy. The underlying issue—and this will sound familiar at this point—is that the insurance industry is literally designed not to benefit patients but instead to benefit shareholders. The entire business model is premised on the idea that denying care, pricing insurance products "aggressively," and even denying coverage are all necessary to keep the industry afloat. No other industrialized country tolerates such an adversarial relationship between actual patients and payors—only in the United States is access to healthcare viewed exclusively through the lens of commerce.

The cost of this is staggering on an individual and a societal level. Consider: in the United States right now, about 13 percent of American adults have no health insurance at all.† This translates into millions of people who are fully exposed to the tremendous costs of our healthcare system. Not surprisingly, these people are more likely to be younger, poorer, or minorities. Is it any wonder that the leading cause of bankruptcy is medical bills? And while it's true that some progress has been made in driving down the number of uninsured thanks to the passage of the Affordable Care Act, a consortium of private and public interests has been working steadily for years to undermine and destroy the protections of the law, meaning the number of uninsured is going up once again.

---

* YouGov. (2017, July 28). While nearly half of all US adult trust insurance companies, most find their language confusing. https://today.yougov.com/topics/finance/articles-reports/2017/07/18/trust-in -insurance.
† Centers for Disease Control and Prevention. Health insurance coverage. https://www.cdc.gov/ nchs/fastats/health-insurance.htm.

For the people who are fortunate enough to have insurance, the picture is only marginally better. This group of people are often afraid to change jobs and lose their insurance, confused by the small print of their plan, severely limited in their treatment options and access to practitioners and medications, and at risk of sky-high medical bills.

This last issue is particularly troubling, and it's a great focusing example of the larger issues plaguing the insurance industry. In a 2020 study published in the prestigious *Journal of American Medical Association*, researchers looked at 350,000 people who had scheduled elective surgery between 2012 and 2017. Unlike emergency medical procedures, where the patient has little or no control over who, when, and where they will need medical care, elective surgeries can be scheduled in advance. This gives people time to make sure their providers are in-network, or that they belong to the insurance coverage pool offered by their carrier. Among this privileged group of patients—having both private insurance and the luxury of time to schedule their procedures—the study authors found that one in five, or 20 percent, still receive "surprise medical bills" after the procedure. These surprise medical bills averaged an extra $2,000 per patient, on top of what the patient already paid in premiums and deductibles.*

How is this possible, even for the most careful patients? The answer lies in the sheer complexity of the medical system. Health insurance companies maintain networks of doctors who are "in network" and base their reimbursement on membership in this network. But even for the largest insurance companies, there are often glaring gaps in their provider networks, and this can be devastating for patients. This is because medicine is a team sport. For example, during an elective surgery, the surgeon might be in-network, but that doesn't mean everyone the patient comes into contact with is, including providers the patient will never meet or see. This includes anesthesiologists, assistants, and other specialists. If these affiliated physicians aren't also in-network, then the policy's rules kick in: the insurance company will reimburse the patient for a small percentage of the out-of-network rate and pass along the rest of the costs to the patient.

If it's this bad for elective procedures with in-network providers, the situation is exponentially worse for true medical emergencies. Nothing illustrates this better than the COVID-19 pandemic that swept through the country in 2020. COVID-19 is the disease caused by the novel coronavirus,

---

* MarketWatch. (2020, February 15). 1 in 5 Americans get hit with a surprise medical bill after elective surgery—here's how much they pay and how to avoid it. https://www.marketwatch.com/story/1-in-5-americans-get-hit-with-a-2000-surprise-medical-bill-after-elective-surgery-study-says-2020-02-12.

which emerged in China sometime in late 2019 and quickly traveled around the world. It's a highly contagious respiratory infection that causes a wide range of symptoms, ranging from mild or nonexistent to lethal. Even as scientists and researchers were racing to better understand the virus and who it affected, millions of Americans tested positive for the virus through the summer of 2020, and the ultimate death toll would exceed half a million people.* While the sheer destructive nature of the virus and the ensuing economic collapse dominated headlines, a lesser-noticed aspect has been attracting attention: sky-high medical bills for patients who are hospitalized.

According to FAIR Health, between 15 and 20 percent of patients who seek treatment for COVID-19 will need to be hospitalized. The average cost of treatment for patients without insurance or with out-of-network providers is $73,300. For patients who see only in-network providers, the average cost is $38,221.† While much of this cost is covered by insurance, the media was full of stories of patients with complex cases who were surprised with six-figure medical bills. Researchers at Johns Hopkins estimated that the average out-of-pocket expenses for COVID-19 in-patient treatment ranged somewhere between $1,700 and $2,200 per patient.‡

The combination of expensive medical care, high premiums, and high deductibles means that Americans are paying obscenely high costs for health coverage. At the top income levels—including the super-rich who can afford private, top-notch, concierge healthcare—this cost may amount to an afterthought. But for most people, even people who are considered middle or upper-middle class, the costs can be crippling. According to the Bureau of Labor Statistics, the percentage of income spent on healthcare for families ranges from a whopping 35 percent of pre-tax income for the lowest income brackets up to 3.5 percent for people in the highest income brackets.§ To put this into perspective, most financial experts recommend that housing should take about 30 percent of the monthly budget. How is it acceptable that poor people are paying more for healthcare than the recommended amount of rent? And once you combine those expenses, it represents 65 percent of monthly expenses—before food, transportation, and utilities are included. And the situation is compounded by the sky-high

---

* Johns Hopkins University. Coronavirus resource center. https://coronavirus.jhu.edu/map.html.

† Fair Health. Costs for a hospital stay for COVID-19. https://www.fairhealth.org/article/costs-for-a-hospital-stay-for-covid-19.

‡ Johns Hopkins University, Coronavirus Resource Center. COVID-19 hospitalizations could mean high out-of-pocket medical costs for many Americans. https://hub.jhu.edu/2020/07/06/out-of-pocket-costs-covid-19-hospitalization/.

§ Advisory Board, (2019,May 2). How much of Americans' paychecks go to health care, charted. https://www.advisory.com/daily-briefing/2019/05/02/health-care-costs.

rate of chronic diseases and obesity at every income bracket. The sicker a person is, the more they spend on healthcare—and the more likely they are to get a surprise medical bill and the higher risk they are for bankruptcy. It's a grim negative feedback loop that many Americans will never escape.

In a very real way, this system actually makes people sicker and worse off. Multiple studies have shown that patients with chronic diseases like diabetes are at much greater risk of suffering from anxiety and/or depression related to the high costs of their medical treatment, whether they have insurance or not.*

Part of this is driven by the advent of high-deductible insurance plans that pass along much of the cost of routine health care to Americans. According to a survey performed by the Kaiser Family Foundation, the average premiums for employer-sponsored health coverage were $20,500 in 2019, with an additional out-of-pocket expense of $6,000. The average deductible for a single covered person was $1,655, while family deductibles of $12,000 are common.†

I have heard too many stories from younger, healthier people being quoted extravagant premiums for basic insurance coverage. In one recent case, a young, healthy man under the age of forty was quoted an annual premium of almost $4,000 for a skimpy insurance plan that wouldn't cover his basic healthcare costs and included a high deductible anyway. With expenses like these, it's no wonder so many younger people skip insurance coverage at all, putting them at risk of an expensive medical event like a car accident that can literally destroy their financial future.

This issue—skipping insurance or delaying care because of cost—isn't limited to young, healthy people. According to a 2019 Gallup poll, one-quarter of Americans have put off getting treatment for a condition because of the cost. This is the highest level ever recorded.‡ When people put off medical care, the result is too often more advanced disease when they do finally get to the doctor, or they may even suffer an acute medical problem like a heart attack or stroke that may have been prevented with adequate medical care at the earlier stage of development.

One of the standard industry responses to complaints about the high cost of medical coverage is to pass along the blame to the hospitals and

---

* Iturralde E, Chi FW, Grant RW, et al. Association of anxiety with high-cost health care use among individuals with type 2 diabetes. *Diabetes Care.* 2019;42(9):1669-1674. doi:10.2337/dc18-1553.

† 2019 Employer Health Benefits Survey. Kaiser Family Foundation. (2019, September 25). https://www.kff.org/health-costs/report/2019-employer-health-benefits-survey/.

‡ Gallup. (2019, December 9). More Americans delaying medical treatment due to cost. https://news.gallup.com/poll/269138/americans-delaying-medical-treatment-due-cost.aspx.

Patient History: The $24,000 Drug

As a practicing medical professional, I've seen too many examples to count of patients who have been mistreated by the insurance and medical industry. In one notable case, I saw a new patient with Crohn's disease. This patient had been seen by a gastroenterologist, who recommended Remicade infusions every eight weeks. Because this drug wasn't included on his formulary, it meant paying $8,000 every quarter, or $24,000 a year. When the patient pushed back, the GI told him there was no other option. The doctor even tried to get authorization through the insurance company's peer-to-peer process but failed. Ultimately, the patient had no choice to pay the price—as far as he was concerned, it was pay or suffer. Sadly, this story happens every day.

---

providers. But this flimsy excuse doesn't withstand even the slightest scrutiny. Just looking at 2018, a picture emerges of an insurance industry that is flush with cash. Consider these industry-wide figures reported by the National Association of Insurance Commissioners:

- In a one-year period, "administrative costs" for insurance companies increased 17.7 percent while premiums increased by 6.5 percent.

- Industry-wide, insurance companies reported an eye-popping income of $24 billion, an almost 50 percent increase over the previous year.*

- Driven by strong profits, since 2014, health insurance stocks have outperformed the Standard & Poor 500 index of stocks by 106 percent.†

Providers Suffer Too

So far, we've concentrated on the payor side of the insurance industry, exposing the financial, emotional, and health toll the industry extracts

---

* National Association of Insurance Commissioners. U.S. health insurance industry: 2018 annual results. https://naic.org/documents/topic_insurance_industry_snapshots_2018_health_ins_ind_report.pdf.

† The Council of Economic Advisers. (2019, March). The profitability of health insurers. https://www.whitehouse.gov/wp-content/uploads/2018/03/The-Profitability-of-Health-Insurance-Companies.pdf.

from ordinary Americans, who are unequipped to push back against companies that literally control their access to health care. But there is another side to the equation as well, and the picture there is equally as grim: the provider side.

The insurance industry, including public insurance like the government behemoth Medicare, has wreaked havoc on the delivery of medical care, thanks to the focus on controlling cost and maximizing profit (excluding Medicare, which doesn't make a profit). The industry has managed to penetrate the most sacred of medical spaces—the patient room—and in many cases warped beyond recognition physicians' ability to practice medicine the way they want to or have been trained to do. This situation has everything to do with the poor job satisfaction and frustration so many doctors feel at work.

Put simply, insurance companies view physicians as the gatekeepers to healthcare and put enormous pressure on doctors to help push costs down. Because the doctors themselves are rarely willing participants in this effort, insurance companies resort to blunt financial bullying to accomplish their goals. And sadly, this effort has been devastatingly effective. In 2018, a nonpartisan trade group called the Alliance for the Adoption of Innovation in Medicine, conducted a survey of six hundred doctors to gauge their views of the insurance industry. A staggering 89 percent of physicians say that don't have "adequate influence" in making patient care decisions. Further, 87 percent directly criticized health insurers for interfering in prescribing treatments.* This interference takes the form of requiring prior authorization before procedures can be performed or prescriptions written, requiring that doctors follow clinical care plans developed by non-medical personnel at the insurance company rather than relying on their own clinical judgement, denying coverage for procedures, and refusing to cover screening tests that might help detect disease earlier. As a result, more than half (52 percent) said they were considering leaving medicine, and more than two-thirds (67 percent) said they wouldn't recommend a career in medicine.

Denying screening tests has a particularly direct and negative effect on patients. Consider just one example: PSA tests in men. The PSA test is designed to measure prostate specific antigen; elevated or rising levels of PSA signal the possible presence of prostate cancer. This is an inexpensive and mostly noninvasive blood test that has been the subject of considerable

---

* Fierce Healthcare. (2018, October, 30). Who's calling the shots? Doctors worry about insurers overriding their treatment decisions. https://www.fiercehealthcare.com/practices/who-s-calling-shots-doctors-worry-insurers-overriding-their-treatment-decisions.

controversy. Before 2012, PSA testing was routine for men over the age of fifty. In 2012, however, the United States Preventive Service Task Force reversed itself and no longer recommended routine PSA screening. As a result, screening was dropped from insurance plans, and PSA screening rates plummeted. Before 2018, PSA testing wasn't recommended for most men, even if it could help catch early cancer. The result was predictable: after years of steadily declining prostate cancer rates, suddenly rates began to climb again.* In response to outcry from patients, in 2018, new guidelines were announced that promoted "shared decision-making" for screening and allowed screening among men who wanted it. As a result, limited coverage for PSA testing was restored in theory if not in practice. Today, Medicare—the largest insurer of older men—covers one PSA screening per year, but there are enough loopholes in the rules that coverage denial for PSA screening is common.†

Once again, these dry numbers mask a slow-moving tragedy. In a real way, men are suffering from these opaque guidelines and shifting rules. It will never be possible to accurately know how many men missed early signs of prostate cancer between 2012 and 2018 and how many men died of their disease. Likewise, there is no data on how the current situation is affecting men's overall health—it will take years of data analysis before some intrepid researcher announces that PSA screening can be an effective tool in identifying and treating prostate cancer, and who knows how many families will suffer between today and that day.

PSA screening is just one example of how this dysfunctional system has real-world consequences—there are plenty more. One of the most frustrating aspects of this is that almost everyone involved in the system knows that something is deeply wrong, but the entrenched interests arguing against reform are powerless against the billion-dollar entities that profit handsomely under the current system.

Writing in the *Washington Post* in late 2019, Dr. William Bennet Jr., a professor of pediatrics at Indiana University School of Medicine, eloquently covered how this looks from a physician's point of view: "As a gastroenterologist, I often prescribe expensive medications or tests for my patients. But for insurance companies to cover those treatments, I must submit a 'prior authorization' to the companies, and it can take days or weeks to hear back. If the insurance company denies coverage, which

---

* American Cancer Society. Cancer statistics center. https://cancerstatisticscenter.cancer.org/#!/cancer-site/Prostate.

† Medpagetoday.com. (2019, August 20). When Medicare stops covering a test without warning. https://www.medpagetoday.com/blogs/kevinmd/81716.

occurs frequently, I have the option of setting up a special type of physician-to-physician appeal called a 'peer-to-peer.'... On most occasions, the peer reviewer is unqualified to make an assessment about the specific services. They usually have minimal or incorrect information about the patient....The insurance company will say this system makes sure patients get the right medications. It doesn't. It exists so that many patients will fail to get the medications they need."[*]

Not only is this personally debilitating for many physicians, it adds layers of administrative complexity. A leading reason many smaller physician practices end up selling their practices to hospital networks is to relieve the administrative burden of dealing with insurance companies that throw up roadblocks at every step of the process. In fact, even doctors who do end up working for hospitals are still spending an incredible amount of time dealing with the paperwork and bureaucratic hoops created by insurance companies. According to the Medscape Physician Compensation Report 2018, which surveyed twenty thousand physicians across thirty specialties, doctors spend a "mind-boggling" amount of time on administrative tasks. Almost a third of these physicians reported spending twenty hours a week on paperwork, most of it related to insurance and documentation. When doctors are spending this much time on paperwork, it's that much less time they can spend focusing on what they're actually trained for: patient care.

And it gets worse. Not only are physicians battling with insurance companies for the right to make medical decisions about their patients, they are actually being told by insurance companies how they can practice medicine. Believe it or not, many managed care companies actually dictate how much time physicians are allowed to spend with patients and still bill for the visit. Typically, doctors are allowed to spend only ten to fifteen minutes with each patient. There is literally no way medicine can be effectively practiced under these circumstances. The key to excellent patient care is often through taking a good history, which is a skill physicians hone over the years. Taking a good history takes time and means asking probing questions to determine what the patient's complaints are, how his or her lifestyle may be related, how various symptoms might be tied together, and obtain a thorough family history. This just isn't possible in ten minutes.

With so many doctors complaining publicly about these rules, what's the rationale behind it? Why would insurance companies feel it necessary

---

[*] Bennet, William Jr. (Washington Post, 2019, October 22). Insurance companies aren't doctors. So why do we keep letting them practice medicine? https://www.washingtonpost.com/opinions/2019/10/22/insurance-companies-arent-doctors-so-why-do-we-keep-letting-them-practice-medicine/.

to impose time limits on patient care? Of course, the answer is related to money. Put simply, the more patients a doctor sees, the more money that doctor can bill. So naturally, time limits on patient care go hand in hand with patient quotas, meaning that insurance companies are actually dictating how many patients a physician must see in a given period. A study in the *Journal of General Internal Medicine* noted that, "Physicians who do not see the number of contractually stipulated patients often earn less and, in some cases, are penalized financially."*

The only reason this is allowed is because patients are already terrified and feel powerless, and the entities that should be protecting patients—especially government entities—have been thoroughly compromised by the financial might of the insurance industry itself. There is no effective patient advocacy in the United States. Even modest changes that would benefit patients are stymied or stifled, and when some reform does finally manage to overcome these systemic obstacles, it is immediately attacked and weakened.

In reality, any rational system would focus on preventative medicine. It would focus on whole-patient care and giving patients the tools to make their own medical decisions and have access to the care they need, before a crisis forces them into a hospital. But there's no chance of the industry policing itself, not with shareholder profit driving decision-making. The only way there will be meaningful patient-centric reform is a mass patient movement. And sadly, the only way patients will be finally empowered to claim their own power is for our whole system to hit rock bottom, causing so much unnecessary illness and economic devastation that millions of patients finally lose their fear of the industry and demand better.

If the insurance companies could just shift their mindset to focusing on prevention, we would actually lower healthcare delivery costs and our patients would be healthier, requiring less testing, less imaging, less follow-up, and ultimately fewer medical bills!

---

* Solomon J. How strategies for managing patient visit time affect physician job satisfaction: a qualitative analysis. *J Gen Intern Med.* 2008;23(6):775-780. doi:10.1007/s11606-008-0596-y.

Chapter 6

The Pharmaceutical Industry

"Hope is beyond price and the pharmaceutical companies, which are run by businessmen not altruists, price their products accordingly."

—**Henry Marsh**

People have been using plants and other natural substances as medicines for millennia, but what we recognize as the modern pharmaceutical industry didn't really arise until the 19th and 20th century. Before it became one of the largest and richest industries in the world, the pharmaceutical industry was pushed forward by enterprising individuals who studied remedies that were often hundreds of years old. One of the most compelling examples of this is the 1783 monograph on digitalis, written by an English doctor named William Withering. Withering discovered that digitalis—actually a toxic extract of the foxglove plant—improved heart function and reduced swelling in the heart muscle. His methods and monograph laid the groundwork for other physicians to explore new medicines over the next century.*

---

* Britannica. Pharmaceutical industry. https://www.britannica.com/technology/pharmaceutical-industry/Isolation-and-synthesis-of-compounds.

Throughout the 19th century, scientists using new methods began to isolate compounds found in medicinal plants. Among the most important of these was morphine (isolated from opium in 1804), quinine (1820), and even cocaine (1860). This ability to isolate individual compounds made it easier to study the effects of these substances on human health and to standardize dosing.*

During this early period, pharmaceutical development really focused on three main areas: vaccine development, pain management, and infectious disease control. This focus made sense in the dangerous world of the 19th century. Prior to the discovery of morphine, ether, and other pain-management drugs, surgeries were excruciating and many patients didn't survive. Similarly, unlike today when largely preventable "lifestyle diseases" like heart disease are the main killers, the biggest killers by far were viruses and bacteria. A look at the earliest "drugs" reads like a who's who of deadly microbes, with a smallpox vaccine showing up in the late 18th century and a vaccine against rabies introduced in 1885.†

But it wasn't until the development of antibiotics that the contours of the modern pharmaceutical industry really emerged. The story most often repeated goes like this: in 1928, English physician Alexander Fleming identified a strain of mold in a petri dish that had incredible anti-bacterial power. Over the next twelve years, the scientific community worked to stabilize and produce penicillin in large enough quantities to test it against various bacteria. Once it was proven to work, Fleming was awarded the Nobel Prize for his work and the age of antibiotics was ushered in, signaling one of the greatest leaps forward in public health in human history.

The actual story, however, is more complicated and shows both the strengths and weaknesses that would emerge in drug development in the coming decades. In fact, the early challenge with penicillin wasn't proving it worked—Fleming himself had demonstrated that early on, and subsequent physicians backed his work up with different strains of penicillin. The early challenge was producing enough penicillin to test and later distribute. From its discovery, penicillin was notoriously difficult to isolate, purify, and stabilize. In the decade after its discovery, scientists at Oxford worked on ways to produce more penicillin, eventually developing a fermentation process that worked. Still, even with a new method, they were

---

* Britannica. Pharmaceutical industry. https://www.britannica.com/technology/pharmaceutical-industry/Isolation-and-synthesis-of-compounds.

† Britannica. Pharmaceutical industry. https://www.britannica.com/technology/pharmaceutical-industry/Isolation-and-synthesis-of-compounds.

only able to create enough penicillin for skimpy clinical trials—certainly not enough to use as an effective medication.

While researchers were working, the imperatives of World War II became increasingly pressing. Shortages of material began to affect their work, even as the need for an antibiotic became a priority. Eventually, the group at Oxford realized they needed help and looked across the Atlantic to America. In this country, the federal government first got involved and developed an improved fermentation process, but it still wasn't enough. Meanwhile, organizers began to plan a massive D-Day invasion of Normandy, meaning that massive quantities of penicillin would be needed to save wounded soldiers. Hoping to scale up production, the government turned to private industry and enlisted companies including Merck, Pfizer, and Squibb to work on the problem. Using their knowledge of mass drug production and fermentation, company researchers quickly developed a way to mass-produce penicillin, and Pfizer soon built the world's first deep fermentation penicillin plant. By the time the soldiers hit the beaches, there was enough penicillin for them—and within two years, around the end of the war—penicillin was widely available for everyone.* The first "wonder drug" had been born.

This is where most histories of penicillin end, but what happened after the war is worth noting. The government stepped back from its active role in antibiotic development, and the private companies took over. Pfizer, in particular, sent representatives all over the world, opening market after market and building plants in far-flung corners of the globe. At the same time, company chemists were testing every mold sample they could find and isolated more antibiotics, including neomycin and erythromycin.† Not only had the age of antibiotics officially begun, we had entered the age of big pharma.

Not surprisingly, the mechanism of government regulation grew up alongside this industry. In 1938, the Federal Food, Drug, and Cosmetic Act gave the Food and Drug Administration the power to regulate the safety of new drugs. The 1945 Penicillin Amendment gave FDA specific jurisdiction over antibiotics. In 1962—after several drug-related scandals including a polio vaccine that caused about two hundred cases of polio and outrage over birth defects caused by thalidomide—Congress passed the Kefauver-Harris Drug Amendments. These amendments were strenuously opposed

---

* American Chemical Society. Discovery and development of penicillin. https://www.acs.org/content/acs/en/education/whatischemistry/landmarks/flemingpenicillin.html
† Wikipedia. Timeline of antibiotics. https://en.wikipedia.org/wiki/Timeline_of_antibiotics.

by the drug companies because they created a new standard: companies had to prove to the FDA that their drugs were effective before they could market them.*

This background is important to understand because these crucial years are when the modern pharmaceutical industry emerged. The story of penicillin is a crowning achievement in human health, and the pharmaceutical companies are quick to remind any skeptics that their products have vastly improved human health. And while that's undeniably true when it comes to vaccines and antibiotics, from the moment the war ended and countries around the world clamored for life-saving antibiotics, profits were the main driver for the rapid global expansion of the drug industry. And from its earliest days, the pharmaceutical industry learned to push back against regulation and oversight with the message that oversight hindered their ability to deliver life-saving medications.

To hear the drug industry tell it, any problems with their products are flukes, and the main problem is the crushing weight of regulation that makes drug discovery so expensive. As of 2019, a study by Tufts University found it cost an average of $2.6 billion to bring a single successful drug to market (this study was disputed, with another group finding the average cost was $900 million, but the pharma companies like this higher figure so I'll give them the benefit of the doubt).† Most of this cost is research and development and includes the cost of the tens of thousands of drugs that fail the rigorous approval process. Once a drug is approved, it's protected by a patent for the next seventeen years, although some of that time is typically lost in the approval process. What this means in practical sense is that pharmaceutical companies have about twelve years to recoup their investment in a new drug before generic companies can mass-produce the drug and offer it at a fraction of the original cost.‡ In effect, this turns drug discovery into a gamble: to profit, companies have to invest in "molecules" that are effective and can withstand the rigorous approval process, then have enough widespread efficacy that the company can recoup its investment before the patent period runs out.

---

* U.S. Food & Drug Administration. Milestones in U.S. food and drug law history. https://www.fda.gov/about-fda/fdas-evolving-regulatory-powers/milestones-us-food-and-drug-law-history.

† Policy & Medicine. A tough road: cost to develop one new drug is $2.6 billion. https://www.policymed.com/2014/12/a-tough-road-cost-to-develop-one-new-drug-is-26-billion-approval-rate-for-drugs-entering-clinical-de.html.

‡ U.S. Food and Drug Administration. Frequently asked questions on patients and exclusivity. https://www.fda.gov/drugs/development-approval-process-drugs/frequently-asked-questions-patents-and-exclusivity#howlongpatentterm.

Looked at this way, the pharmaceutical industry operates a high-wire act with swashbuckling daring, placing billion-dollar bets on drug development and wagering on their ability to dramatically improve human health. And if this was how things operated in the real world, the drug companies would deserve all of the accolades and moral praise they regularly claim as their own. But let's step back and get some perspective here. According to the industry's lobbying and trade group, the all-powerful Pharmaceutical Research and Manufacturers Association (PhRMA), the biopharmaceutical industry in the United States alone has a yearly economic impact of $1.3 *trillion*. This one industry accounts for about 4 percent of the total U.S. economic output.* And remember the scrappy pharmaceutical companies that helped develop penicillin and spread it around the world? They're not so little anymore. Pfizer now boasts annual revenues more than $51 billion. Other top players in the pharmaceutical industry include Roche ($50 billion in annual revenue), Novartis ($47 billion in annual revenue), Merck ($46 billion in annual revenue) and GlaxoSmithKline ($43 billion in annual revenue). Together the top-ten companies generate $392.5 billion in annual revenue.†

These eye-popping sums create a financial incentive that cannot be denied. Today, the pharmaceutical industry is represented by one of the most lavishly funded lobbying groups (PhRMA) and has managed to twist the drug approval and distribution market almost entirely to its own advantage—and almost entirely to the disadvantage of the patients who rely on its products to stay alive. How is this possible? It's accomplished through several mechanisms, most of which the general public is unaware of. These include a corrupted FDA approval process, powerful lobbying efforts that are designed to protect and consolidate industry control while stifling government efforts to reduce drug prices, a patronage system that pressures physicians to prescribe and warps insurance formularies, intensive direct-to-consumer advertising programs, and finally a highly sophisticated and relentless public relations effort to discredit so-called alternative therapies and frighten consumers.

And all of this is hidden behind a veil of strict secrecy. Pharmaceutical company executives and researchers are frequently bound by non-disclosure agreements that prevent them from talking about their work. I know

---

* Select USA. Biopharmaceutical spotlight.. https://www.selectusa.gov/pharmaceutical-and-bio-tech-industries-united-states#:~:text=The%20overall%20economic%20impact%20of,U.S.%20 output%20in%202015%20alone.
† Becker's Hospital Review. Top 10 pharma companies by revenue. https://www.beckershospitalre-view.com/pharmacy/top-10-pharma-companies-by-revenue.html.

for a fact that research and development employees for these big companies can never, under any circumstance, discuss anything they are working on! If these companies are here to help people and advance the medical community, then all this information (pitfalls and success) should be shared with others in the industry so they don't waste time/energy. There should be a more synergistic approach to helping advance pharma if they really cared about the good of the people. What they shouldn't be doing is mandating that their employees are sworn to secrecy in an effort to prevent other pharma companies from profiting.

The FDA: Part of the Problem

Many of the problems with the drug industry begin with the FDA approval process itself—a process that was designed to ensure only safe and well-vetted drugs reach the market. In fact, pharmaceutical money has warped every part of this process, with sometimes disastrous results. From the clinical studies that are required as part of the approval process to the funding of the FDA's regulatory process itself, pharmaceutical companies have created a system that is better at excluding competition than it is at approving drugs. Here are just a few of the strategies they use to accomplish this:

- **Burying bad studies, or even faking or misinterpreting results**. This is the easiest and best way to get a drug approved: just don't report negative results or kill studies early on that are returning questionable results. Believe it or not, this is actually standard operating procedure. Even after a 2015 initiative called AllTrials was set up to advocate that all clinical trials are included, less than half of pharma companies have any policies protecting the integrity of their clinical studies.* This fundamental flaw can have life-or-death consequences. In the 1990s, pharmaceutical giant Merck skewed the results of studies for a COX-2 inhibitor called Vioxx (a highly popular anti-inflammatory drug). The effort to cook the books went so far as actually

---

* Dr. Rath Health Foundation. How the trillion dollar a year pharmaceutical industry rigs the results of its studies. https://www.dr-rath-foundation.org/2017/10/how-the-trillion-dollar-a-year -pharmaceutical-industry-rigs-the-results-of-its-studies/.

ghostwriting clinical results internally and then paying doctors to have the fraudulent studies published under their own names. The result? Vioxx was approved despite evidence that it also caused an increase in heart attack risk. In 2004, after Vioxx was pulled from the market, an official in the FDA's Office of Drug Safety estimated that the use of Vioxx had resulted in fifty-five thousand premature deaths from heart attack and stroke.*

- **Paying researchers and scientists to conduct positive studies.** In an ideal world, scientists would be free of corrupting influences while they carried out the studies we rely on to ensure drugs are safe and effective. In fact, pharma companies have created a patronage system with the leading research universities and institutions that enmeshes supposedly "neutral" researchers in a financial web. This patronage used to be more direct—cash payments or luxury gifts funneled directly to the doctors. Today, it takes the form of honoraria or lavishly funded appointments to corporate advisory boards.† The result are studies and recommendations that are skewed in favor of the drug companies. In one memorable example, in a 2015 paper in *The Lancet*, a group of researchers recommended wider use of hypertensive medications. It later turned out that almost all of the study's authors were financially connected to the companies making the drugs they were recommending. ‡

- **Directly funding the FDA's approval process.** This is a classic case of the fox being in the henhouse. In response to budget shortages at the FDA that caused long drug-approval times, in 1992, Congress passed a law that partly funded the FDA through "user fees" charged to the pharmaceutical companies that were submitting drugs for review. This practice grew quickly, and by 2020, the pharmaceutical industry provided about half of the FDA's overall budget and more than 75 percent of the budget

---

* Union of Concerned Scientists. (2017,October 12). Merck manipulated the science about the drug Vioxx. https://www.ucsusa.org/resources/merck-manipulated-science-about-drug-vioxx#:~:text= Scientists%20from%20the%20pharmaceutical%20giant,patients'%20risk%20of%20heart%20attack.

† Dr. Rath Health Foundation. How the trillion dollar a year pharmaceutical industry rigs the results of its studies. https://www.dr-rath-foundation.org/2017/10/how-the-trillion-dollar-a-year -pharmaceutical-industry-rigs-the-results-of-its-studies/.

‡ Dr. Rath Health Foundation. How the trillion dollar a year pharmaceutical industry rigs the results of its studies. https://www.dr-rath-foundation.org/2017/10/how-the-trillion-dollar-a-year -pharmaceutical-industry-rigs-the-results-of-its-studies/.

devoted to drug approvals. This makes it the only federal agency that is mostly supported by the very same industry it's supposed to be regulating (this is an incredibly powerful statement and I am wondering if it should be a side bar or stand out more on the page). The results? Drugs like nuplazid and uloric that are rushed through the system in response to industry pressure and with deadly results. Both of these drugs were green-lighted despite data showing increased risk of serious side effects and even death.*

The fact that the drug approval process is so fundamentally and dangerously flawed is no accident—it's only part of a larger picture in which the pharmaceutical industry gets to write its own rules or crush measures that might actually benefit patients but conflict with their bottom lines. This is possible because of the vast might of the pharmaceutical lobbying organization, PhRMA. In fact, the pharmaceutical industry is the single biggest lobbying force in Washington. Every year, pharma companies funnel more than $225 million dollars into lobbying efforts. This includes setting up "consumer advocacy" organizations with high-minded–sounding names that are really just fronts for the drug industry.

Although it seems like a lot of money, this is a good investment for the industry. After all, it's the reason drug prices in the United States remain persistently high, why so many ideas for reform are killed immediately, including drug re-importation from foreign markets and bills that would give Medicare the power to negotiate drug prices. The industry's standard playbook is brutally simple but effective: invent some bogus safety claim, and then flood the zone with money, looking for that friendly senator to block the legislation or the committee chairperson willing to bottle it up. The truly sad thing is, this is all done in public and has serious real-world consequences both financially and in terms of human health. But when facing down a trillion-dollar industry with unlimited resources and a political class hooked on that money, what can any single person or poorly funded patient advocacy organization do? Drug reform is truly David versus Goliath, except that Goliath wins this time.

An excellent example of how this system affects patients is the way hospital formularies are warped by the pharmaceutical industry. Hospital formularies—or the lists of drugs that hospitals use for particular

---

* ProPublica. (2018, June 26). FDA Repays Industry by Rushing Risky Drugs to Market. https://www.propublica.org/article/fda-repays-industry-by-rushing-risky-drugs-to-market.

conditions—are supposed to be developed by controlling boards within a hospital and based on the best available evidence of efficacy. In fact, formularies are often manipulated by the many players in the drug pipeline, including pharmacy benefit managers (PBMs) and pharmaceutical companies. These companies have a vested interest in including only the most expensive drugs on a formulary, so they use tactics like discounting some drugs in exchange for including other, more lucrative drugs on the formulary.* By the time a patient is prescribed one of these drugs in the hospital, the fix is already in. And it hardly matters when companies are caught committing this type of fraud—the legal bills are little more than a pesky annoyance.

The same thing happens in private practice with primary care providers (PCPs). PCPs often want to prescribe a certain drug only to find out that the drug is not listed on the patient's insurance formulary, which results in the patient paying astronomical fees for a drug the doctor is recommending! Sometimes the doctor is notified that the drug they want to use is not covered on the patient's insurance formulary, so the patient goes back to the doctor and says, "I can't afford the drug you prescribed," asking for an alternative that may be covered. This forces the PCP to go with a second, less effective option, and ultimately the patient never gets better or improves!

In some cases, PCPs will go to bat for patients. What this means in reality is spending countless hours arguing with the insurance company and completing a prior-authorization to justify to a non-medical insurance company employee why this drug is medically necessary. It is customary for PCPs and their staffs to spend more than twenty-five hours a week arguing with insurance companies about non-formulary or non-covered options for patients. This unnecessary work adds to the already busted-at-the-seams workload for our PCPs and increases costs all around. This isn't even to mention the unfathomable scenario that a non-medically trained person from an insurance company is making a judgment on which medical therapy a PCP may or may not use. And forget about trying to get a more alternative or natural medical option covered by insurance! There are a plethora of alternative medical options, but insurance companies will always deny usage of these approaches because they have not been tested and FDA approved, but remember who is in charge of that process....

---

* Constantine Cannon. Pharmaceutical fraud. https://constantinecannon.com/practice/whistle blower/whistleblower-types/healthcare-fraud/pharmaceutical-fraud/.

How Ads Warp Patients

Unfortunately, all of this is basically treated as an open secret in the medical industry. That's one of the truly shocking things about the corruption of the pharmaceutical industry—most of this is practiced in the open and reported regularly in the media. But these aren't the types of issues that can galvanize the public. Who among us has the time and energy to unravel the byzantine ways the pharmaceutical industry has corrupted its own business and profiteers from sick patients? Who has a voice loud enough to be heard over the amplified roar of the public relations mythology funded by the industry itself?

If most people stop to think about the pharmaceutical industry at all, it's most likely because they are worried about their health and looking for a cure. And guess who would give people that idea? Once again, the pharmaceutical industry is only too happy to step up and fill the void with a tidal wave of powerful messaging, this time through the ubiquitous ads for their products that fill magazines, the Internet, and airwaves.

The industry practice of direct-to-consumer advertising (DTCA) almost ironically was born out of the patients' rights movement. Through the 1980s and early 1990s, consumer advertising for drugs was limited and tightly regulated. At the time, even pharmaceutical executives were opposed to a practice they considered dangerous, as it could infringe on the doctor/patient relationship and potentially confuse patients.* Throughout the 1990s, however, a few powerful forces came together to weaken the FDA resolve against DTCA, including the patient empowerment movement and the beginnings of the movement toward shared decision-making. Patients' rights groups were pushing for more information to be shared with patients. In 1997, the FDA finally submitted and issued rules that opened the floodgate to DTCA.

Once opened, the gates would not close. Well-funded pharmaceutical companies that had once avoided DTCA began pouring tens of millions of dollars into TV ads for their products. Between 1993, before the new FDA rule, and 2005, the amount of spending for DTCA increased from

---

* Donohue J. A history of drug advertising: the evolving roles of consumers and consumer protection. *Milbank Q.* 2006;84(4):659-699. doi:10.1111/j.1468-0009.2006.00464.x.

$166 million (which was mostly PR campaigns) to a staggering $4.2 billion.* Overall, DTCA comprised about 40 percent of all drug marketing that year. By 2016, it had surged to $9.6 billion.†

On the surface, it seems like providing more information to patients would be a good thing—but that's not what's happening here. Instead of empowering patients, the role of DTCA is to transform *patients* into *consumers*. The goal is to convince patients to go into their doctors' offices and request certain medications, whether they're for erectile dysfunction, hair loss, cholesterol management, or so-called lifestyle diseases. Unfortunately, this advertising only has the appearance of oversight and brushes past complicated concepts in medicine that consumers may not understand well, including misrepresenting clinical trials and employing very precise language to mislead patients. At the same time, according to Dr. Robert Shmerling, the senior editor of Harvard Health Publishing, DTCA promotes drugs before their long-term safety is known (remember Vioxx?) and overall raises the cost of medical care as physicians increase prescriptions in response to patient pressure.‡ He cited this scenario relays a lack of complete information, misleading language and claims, and the push to encourage patients to ask for medications they don't need. Pharma companies are essentially fostering a mindset that patients can "take a pill and the problem will go away," instead of helping patients focusing on making deeper changes in combination with less costly and dangerous adjunctive therapies.

The push to transform patients into pharmaceutical consumers wouldn't be complete without a corresponding push to eliminate competition. After all, DTCA only works if consumers believe the drug being promoted is the best (and maybe only) solution for a health concern. In practical terms, this means discrediting any alternative treatments or even downplaying healthy lifestyle changes that could accomplish the same thing—you've probably heard the words, "When diet and exercise isn't enough…" in a pharma ad before.

When it comes to alternative treatments that might threaten their bottom line, pharmaceutical companies can be relentless. This makes sense

* Donohue J. A history of drug advertising: the evolving roles of consumers and consumer protection. *Milbank Q.* 2006;84(4):659-699. doi:10.1111/j.1468-0009.2006.00464.x.

† ScienceDaily, (2019, January 8). Medical marketing has skyrocketed in the past two decades, while oversight remains limited. https://www.sciencedaily.com/releases/2019/01/190109170637.htm.

‡ Harvard Health Publishing. (2019, November 25). Harvard Health Ad Watch: What you should know about direct-to-consumer ads. https://www.health.harvard.edu/blog/harvard-health-ad-watch-what-you-should-know-about-direct-to-consumer-ads-2019092017848.

when you consider that the entire philosophical foundation of alternative and functional medicine is starkly opposed to the philosophy that drives the pharmaceutical industry. In modern pharmaceuticals, companies chose man-made, non-native "molecules" that have specific action against a highly targeted disease or condition. In this way of thinking, "one disease, one drug" means that there are one or more drugs that can be deployed like precision missiles against disease. If those drugs have unpleasant side effects, other drugs can be prescribed to handle those, and so on.

This brings on a phenomena we call "poly pharmacy." This is an actual diagnosis that a doctor may give a patient. It means the patient is on so many drugs their health is impacted. You know there is a problem when you need to prescribe a medicine to help control side effects from another medicine….Where does this madness end?!

There is little or no concern for the whole patient or encouraging treatments or lifestyle changes that can address the underlying conditions that created the disease. Instead, people are viewed as disjointed collections of organs and symptoms that can be treated individually, with little effect on other organs except the occasional side effect. There is no awareness or recognition of how complex our bodies are and how much interaction there is between organ systems. Quite often, medications prescribed by a specialist for one condition in one organ system causes side effects in another organ system. There is a significant failure by many practitioners to recognize the impacts of drugs on other organ systems. As an example, a gastroenterologist may want to prescribe a drug for Crohn's disease but fail to appreciate the effects this drug may have on bone density. Or how a psychiatrist may want to prescribe a drug for major depressive disorder or anxiety but ignore the well-known and published side effects of weight gain and negative hormone effects.

By contrast, functional medicine views a person as a whole, with dozens and dozens of carefully balanced biological systems, chemical reactions, and interactions that all work together to support health. In this approach, pharmaceuticals may sometimes be necessary, but they are the sledgehammers of last resort or they are used in combination with adjunctive therapies to optimize short- and long-term success! There are times and places where these pharmaceuticals are necessary, but they should rarely be the first option. Realistically, many other options should be tried before resorting to synthetic pharmaceutical drugs!

In fact, working in partnership with insurance companies, these so-called "alternative" treatments are discounted as quackery or a waste of money and time. But a quick search of PubMed is revealing. Even without

Dealing with Cancer Doctors

Cancer is challenging enough to deal with for patients, so it's infuriating that many patients also have to deal with close-minded oncologists who refuse to consider therapies that might help their patients. Over the years, I've had many conversations with oncologists who dismiss "alternative" treatments out of hand or—even worse—actively work to convince patients they're dangerous.

A perfect example of this is bioidentical hormone therapy for breast cancer survivors. Under the right circumstances, this therapy is perfectly safe and has measurable benefits for women. Unfortunately, in case after case, traditional oncologists tell these women if they go on bioidentical hormones they're going to get cancer again and kill themselves, even if the cancer has been clear for ten-plus years. For these doctors, the symptoms that prompted the patient to start bioidentical hormone therapy in the first place are meaningless as they push to prevent women from a perfectly safe therapy. Yet once again, these conventionally trained oncologists do not look at the patient as a whole and neglect the well-known total body-aging effects of woman who don't have healthy hormone levels after cancer treatment. With anything in medicine, we need to calculate the risk versus the reward, and it's a well-known fact of how influential healthy hormone levels are for our bodies, so does the risk of a woman not having healthy hormone levels (and expediting the aging process) outweigh the undocumented risk of cancer recurrence in woman using bioidentical hormones? In most cases, I think not! You can even argue the fact that individuals who have successfully beat cancer are at a higher risk for cancer recurrence if they don't use bioidentical hormones. As I mentioned early, individuals who don't maintain healthy hormone levels have their bodies age MUCH faster, and if this happens, then the individual may be at higher risk for cancer recurrence.

the extraordinary level of funding enjoyed by conventional medications, there are thousands of studies validating alternative approaches. Just like their conventional counterparts, physicians who prescribe alternative medicines are relying on a rich body of high-quality evidence validating their approach. But somehow, through brute repetition and tactics that rely on fear, this entire body of evidence is dismissed as unreliable, fraudulent, and even dangerous.

The irony here is that the charges leveled against alternative medicine are actually the issues that plague pharmaceuticals. In a case of massive projection, the evidence that supports some of the biggest drugs has turned out to be unreliable, fraudulent, and even dangerous. The very same criticisms the industry uses to undermine its "competition" are better aimed at the industry itself.

To avoid quacks, look for the science. There should be double-blind, pla-cebo-controlled, gold standard studies to back up everything I recommend to patients. I don't get pushback from patients. I get it from their doctors. A lot of them don't read anything after they graduate.

—Elyse Marrone, Clinical Director
Lifestyle Nutrition Institute

Unfortunately, without a revolution in medicine, it looks like the future holds more of the same. The pharmaceutical industry isn't getting less powerful; the standards and systems we rely on to approve medications aren't being reinforced and reformed. Worse, they are being stretched and weakened even more. This was clearly seen during the 2020 COVID-19 pandemic, when drugs and vaccines were authorized by the FDA under "emergency use authorization" for mass use in the population during uncertain times. Here's the FDA language describing this status:

The Emergency Use Authorization (EUA) authority allows FDA to help strengthen the nation's public health protections against chemical, biological, radiological, and nuclear (CBRN) threats, including infectious diseases, by facilitating the availability and use of medical countermeasures (MCMs) needed during public health emergencies.

Under section 564 of the Federal Food, Drug, and Cosmetic Act (FD&C Act), when the Secretary of HHS declares that an emergency use authorization is appropriate, FDA may authorize unapproved medical products or unapproved uses of approved medical products to be used in an emergency to diagnose, treat, or prevent serious or life-threatening diseases or conditions caused by CBRN threat agents when certain criteria are met, including there are no adequate, approved, and available alternatives. The HHS declaration to support such use must be based on one of four types of determinations of threats or potential threats by the Secretary of HHS, Homeland Security, or Defense.

So we helped the public by administering something that may not be safe and has not been tested fully? How does that make any sense? Or do they not care if it works or not, so they can just work on developing something else to save us from these EUA drugs, vaccines, or procedures?!

The urgency and rush to develop a COVID-19 vaccine made any already stretched set of regulations even more bendy! The race to come to market for the first COVID-19 vaccine was on, and these emergency-use drugs and vaccines very quickly proved to be a product of a rushed and dangerous system as early vaccines were linked to blood clots, intensifying symptoms, and uncertainty (rightfully so).

With hundreds of billions of dollars on the line, the industry will never reform itself. It will take the collective voice of tens of millions of patients—informed patients—to demand something better, something closer to dignity in healthcare. Only when regular people start to demand that they are whole people, not random collections of organs that produce cash, will Americans get the healthcare they deserve.

Chapter 7

How Does This Affect Us?

"America's healthcare system is neither healthy, caring, nor a system."

—Walter Cronkite

It's easy to get overwhelmed by the state of our healthcare system. Over the years, we've seen attempt after attempt at reform fail, often blocked by elements of the healthcare system itself that are concerned about losing lucrative profits or not understanding the operational efficiencies of nonmedical politicians. At the same time, on a national level, we've been losing ground as everything from overall mortality to obesity rates to the cost of health insurance for families continues to skyrocket. Clearly, patients are not winning or reaping any benefit, which is shocking coming from the planet's wealthiest and most intellectually advanced country!

If there were an easy fix, that would be great—but this is a complex issue that has taken decades to develop and touches every American's life in some way. And the scale of the problem is enormous. It's not only that the insurance industry profiteers, or that medical schools are pushing too many doctors into specialties while hospitals are consolidating into huge health networks with in-house doctors, or that the pharmaceutical company's trillions have corrupted the prescription drug market, or the fact that patients can't understand their health or aren't empowered to make more informed decisions. It's all of these things. All of these failed individual systems are linked together (just like our organ systems are only as good as their weakest link!).

But it's how this affects individuals that matters most. None of us are a collection of statistics or policy positions, which means there is NO one-size-fits-all medicine and we cannot be treated the same! Each of us is unique and invested in staying healthy and keeping our loved ones healthy, so why is our healthcare system not? Why isn't a system designed to be compassionate sympathetic to our needs and goals? We all want to know that if we get sick, we'll get good information from our healthcare providers so we can make good decisions about what to do next. Decisions that are based on good science and what's really best for patients. More importantly, we want to know what we can do to preserve and protect health, to prevent disease in the first place and focus on slowing the aging process. This means we need good information.

The more tragic effect of the problems with our healthcare system is what it does to individuals and how it affects our decision-making process. People aren't empowered to invest in themselves or their health, while practitioners are bullied into following templated treatment protocols and formulary drug schemes and incentivized financially by patient volume quotas. We don't have adequate time to educate our patients on their health or work or lifestyle factors to help patients take control of their own health. Instead, many patients just do what their doctors dictate or their insurance company tells them is the cheapest or only option available. They only schedule doctors' appointments according to their insurance's plan and only take the drugs covered by their plan, without understanding that these rules weren't written because they make people healthier. They were written to ensure that patients could get the bare minimum in care without bankrupting an insurance company. For most people, one of the first questions that comes up when they fall sick or need care is, "How much will this cost? Is it covered?"

This is wrong. No one should think this way, either patients or doctors. This is why the healthcare system never improves—we need to change the mindset of patients as well as the practitioners who are forced to practice in certain ways in order to keep the doors open.

Instead of staying healthy, cost is the primary driver for healthcare decisions. This is compounded by confusion over how "the system" works. Talk to any cancer patient about their treatment, and it quickly becomes obvious how overwhelming and expensive treatment is. Or talk to the average American and ask if they know what their blood test results mean. Patients don't need to have complex diseases to be confused. Plenty of day-to-day, average patients have no idea how to interpret their own health.

Yet tragically, this is accepted as "normal." One common piece of advice for cancer patients is to find an advocate to help them deal with their insurance company and care teams. The assumption behind this advice is that cancer patients are too depleted (physically and mentally) by their treatment to spend the hours on the phone arguing about which treatments and which specialists are in-network and covered. But take a step back and really think about that: our system is so damaged that the sickest among us—people whose lives truly do depend on getting good healthcare—are told it's almost impossible to navigate the system while in treatment. Is that right? What about the people who don't have the luxury of a well-informed advocate? Or don't have a spouse or any family or friends to support them? Can they rely on this system, or do they just fall victim to a broken system more quickly?

The reality is that everyone is trapped in this same system, including the doctors who struggle to deliver the best care they can (keep in mind this is a direct violation of that Hippocratic oath to do no harm). Money and time are the biggest influences, and ultimately the system is designed to deter people from trying to fight it. Its complexity is actually a defense mechanism that protects revenue and profit behind a wall of complexity. It's hard enough for highly educated patients to figure it out—it's that much harder for people with less education or people who are working sixty-plus hours a week to support themselves and their families. The system is programmed to fail, because failure works for the business model.

The failure of the system extends beyond the hospital walls and into the way people interact with healthcare information today—and where do they get it from. Ask almost any doctor and he or she will tell you that "Dr. Google" or "WebMD" is a serious problem in their practices. Patients without medical training go online to search their condition and find an ocean of disinformation. Some of it comes from scammers who prey on people's ignorance to profit. But some of it also comes from conventional medical sources that are invested in protecting the existing system. In fact, the entrenched interests you've been reading about so far actually benefit from the confusion—anything that disorients patients leaves them feeling more vulnerable and confused is good for them, because what do we do when we are unsure? That's right—we do nothing!

But there is good information out there, and it can make a huge difference in patient's lives and medical care. As an example, let's look at the most common way people interact with the medical system: their annual check-ups. According to most insurance plans, patients are entitled to one "well visit" with their doctor every year. But here's a good question: where's the data showing that one visit a year to the doctor yields the best outcomes for patients? Where are the studies demonstrating what should happen during the annual visit to ensure patients are fully protected and have all the knowledge they need to make their best health decisions?

By this point, you shouldn't be surprised to find out there isn't any such data. In fact, the once-a-year visit and what happens during them has nothing to do with patient care and everything to do with the bottom lines of the insurance companies. It turns out that preventive medicine doesn't really turn much of a profit for insurance companies. The same goes for screening tests. The end result is that these appointments tend to be short and unsatisfying, with no prophylactic education or discussions on preventive medicine, supplements, or slowing down the aging process. There's no focus on health—only on waiting for a condition to get serious enough to warrant a prescription.

In truth, one visit to the doctor every year is not nearly enough, even for healthy and active twenty-five-year-olds. No matter a patient's age, the human body can make clinically significant hormonal, chemical, and physiologic changes in as little time as ninety days (in some areas of the body, in as little as two weeks!). Ideally, we want to detect markers early so we can halt the disease and inflammatory progression, not wait for the disease to gain momentum and present at more severe stages.

This means we need screening tests and more routine examinations, but the rhythm of screening tests is dictated by standards that are set by medical organizations. This includes cholesterol screening, hypertension screening, and tests like the PSA test for men or mammography for women. In a broad sense, these screening tools are invaluable and it's critical to use and interpret them correctly. But unfortunately, thanks to deficiencies in medical education and pressure from insurance companies to reduce costly testing, these screening tests are not being executed and/or interpreted like they should, which limits their value.

For many tests, like cholesterol levels, nutrient levels, and hormones, the reference ranges are way too broad and generalized to make good decisions. If the tests are run in the frequency that we need them in order to accurately assess trends and patterns, then we run into the second problem: gargantuan reference ranges that allow early changes to go undetected by practitioners. These subtle sub-optimal levels may look as though they are in the normal range, but in fact are the earliest indicator of the body changing and very likely are signaling serious underlying problems. And because a patient may only be screened once or twice a year, despite the fact that markers change daily and weekly, those screenings don't give either the patient or the healthcare provider enough information in the right timeframe to intervene.

The conventional medicine mindset is that as long as everything looks like it's within the "normal" range and there are few symptoms, there won't be a diagnosis. In six months, during another ten-minute wellness screening, another screen will be taken as if somehow it's possible to make decisions based on two screens months apart, based on reference ranges that are almost useless. It turns out the accepted reference ranges themselves are also an issue. They are developed from individuals ranging in age from twenty to eighty, making them too vague and generalized to be of much specific use.

So, what's the alternative?

One of the really unfortunate aspects of this issue is that the alternative is obvious. All we need to do is actually listen to the science and practice medicine that's focused on the patient, instead of getting wrapped up in endless calls with insurance companies or pushing back on misinformation. A twice-annual screening can't detect the subtle cellular changes that have no symptoms but that underlie the actual disease process—and in many cases, younger patients who are already experiencing changes that may lead to disease in later years don't even go to the doctor at all. Perhaps worst of all, the typical wellness visit doesn't even look for factors that we know signal worsening health. The standard blood test is totally inadequate, especially if it's only given once or twice a year. For preventive medicine, there aren't nearly enough screens to catch everything.

How can we be so sure this is true? Because there are literally thousands upon thousands of high-quality studies exploring this issue, and there is widespread agreement among healthcare practitioners that disease doesn't just start when a patient experiences a symptom. The earliest detectors of disease are inflammation markers. These show up in the blood as elevated C-reactive protein (CRP), plasma viscosity (PV), homocysteine, and erythrocyte sedimentation rate (ESR), among other inflammatory markers that can help us identify incipient cardiac disease, gastrointestinal issues, metabolic disorders, and many others—long before there are symptoms and while it's still early enough to reverse the underlying disease process and prevent long-term, permanent damage to organs and cells.

While there is hopeful progress that younger doctors are learning to correctly use and interpret more advanced testing, there is still so much needed progress on screening. Patients should be screened more often, with a wider range of tools than what is currently happening. The reference ranges on some of the most common blood tests we use to identify risks need to be brought into alignment with the science. Even the way studies are conducted needs to be changed. In many cases, reference ranges are calculated based on studies performed on people with very different health concerns. How can a twenty-year-old study participant and an eighty-year-old study participant have anything in common, when their health status and needs are dramatically different?

At the most basic level, we need to start considering patients as whole people once again. In a way, this is going back to the "old time" way of practicing medicine and moving away from the push toward sub-sub-sub-specialties. And while there are tremendous obstacles to reorienting medicine to focus on patients—medical education, the rise of massive health networks, and insurance and pharmaceutical industry profiteering—there is actually one collective force that is more powerful than all of them: patients.

The revolution in medicine will come from the bottom up. This is why it's critical to teach patients both about the issues with the current system, but also about the reality of a better way to practice medicine. If there are enough patients calling for change, it will happen. There can be a true shift—and in many ways, this is already happening. Over the last few decades, a new type of patient has emerged. This new patient is educated and hyper-vigilant about their own care. They read about medical care and know what questions to ask to prevent disease, and if diagnosed with a condition, they insist on working with their healthcare provider to develop a treatment plan.

This is happening more out of necessity than anything else—once patients realize the insurance industry and conventional healthcare have failed them, they have to educate themselves. It's not uncommon in our offices for patients to show up after frustrating and ineffective experiences with "conventional" doctors that didn't offer adequate treatment. By the time this patient walks through our door, he or she has often spent a great deal of time and money learning about their own health.

When Dr. Google Meets Youth Marketing

Unfortunately, this movement toward patient education comes with a few caveats. It turns out Dr. Google is a pretty lousy physician. The Internet is swarming with health information, some of it good, some of it unreliable, and much of it based on scams and outright quackery. Anyone on the Internet can say anything, making it confusing for patients and limiting their progress. From a practical point of view, this means healthcare providers are obligated to spend some extra time with each patient to help them sort through all the things they may have read and actually get good information. In a conventional setting—where a physician may be operating under a quota and have only a few minutes with each patient—this more leisurely exchange of information is almost impossible.

The other danger posed by this flood of information is thanks to larger cultural forces and the imperatives of marketing. We live in a youth-obsessed culture that's focused mostly on outer beauty. It used to be fashionable to complain about how ads only depicted beautiful, young people, but in today's more complex, information-saturated Internet culture, it goes so much deeper than that. Social media "influencers"—almost always attractive young people—are paid huge sums to promote products and ideas, often without disclosing their relationship to the advertiser. At the same time, many of these people spend huge amounts of money on cosmetic surgeries or even Photoshop to maintain their own illusion of youth and beauty, and of course they often directly deny this when pressed.

The idea behind all of this is straightforward: you too can look like this, live this life, if you just buy our product. Unfortunately, knowing it's true intellectually does nothing to reduce the strong emotional imperative that youth and beauty are always possible with just one more product, one more prescription, one more therapy.

People are exposed to this false hope constantly. Feel your best. Look your best. Athletes and models are portrayed as mythical creatures that patients can transform into. Every drug ad talks about looking better, feeling better, and reversing a diagnosis. They are designed to lure patients into a healthcare setting. But this is false hope. Drugs don't reverse conditions. People will use their little bit of time and money and won't get results. And, of course, no one reads the side effects inserts before they go into their physician asking for a drug they saw in an ad. It's a no-win situation for consumers, who are vulnerable to scammers, both in conventional and integrative healthcare.

The solution here is to create truly educated patients. From a healthcare provider's perspective, this usually means taking the time to start their healthcare education correctly. It means helping people understand what's really happening with their bodies, how they change over time, and what that means at every stage of life and health. It means dispelling the layered misinformation around topics like diet and nutrition, exercise, disease prevention, and management of chronic conditions. It means giving people the basic tools in health literacy they'll need to go out into the world and continue their own education. If patients can understand the basic science, they can understand the medicine. Healthcare providers need to start on the patients' wavelength and help them understand why their bodies are so complex and why they're aging. If patients can understand this, they will be empowered to make good health choices.

Even better, they'll learn to make healthy choices that are unique to them. This idea that all people need the same things at the same times in their life is ludicrous. Every patient is unique, and all of us experience aging differently. There is no "magic" diet that will work for everyone. If you discover you do better with one style of eating, there's likely a reason for that and you should continue eating that way. It's pointless to compare yourself to other people or worry about what the latest fad diet is.

Along with giving people education, the final step in making the shift to creating autonomous patients is giving them the tools to use that education. This can take many forms, but it's crucial. It means recommending high-quality supplements that have been rigorously tested to contain the ingredients on their labels and that are effective. The supplement market is lightly regulated and full of dubious claims that have only served to make people suspicious. This is unfortunate, because supplementation should be part of almost any personal health plan.

It also means giving people the tools they need to monitor their own health. Patients can learn how to read and use a glycemic index chart. They can use a home-based blood pressure monitor. Patients should be empowered to visit practitioners who are practicing medicine the right way, and it should be very easy to identify the scammers from those who genuinely care. A good integrative medicine practitioner should give patients the tools necessary to have success on their health journey!

At its heart, this is what integrative medicine really is all about, and it will be the focus of the rest of this book. Integrative medicine is the alternative to the chaos and corruption of conventional medicine, as we seek to create educated and empowered patients who are fully in control of their own health and understand what's happening and why. This is truly patient-centered medicine, and it needs to happen now!

PART TWO
A NEW APPROACH

COMPASSION

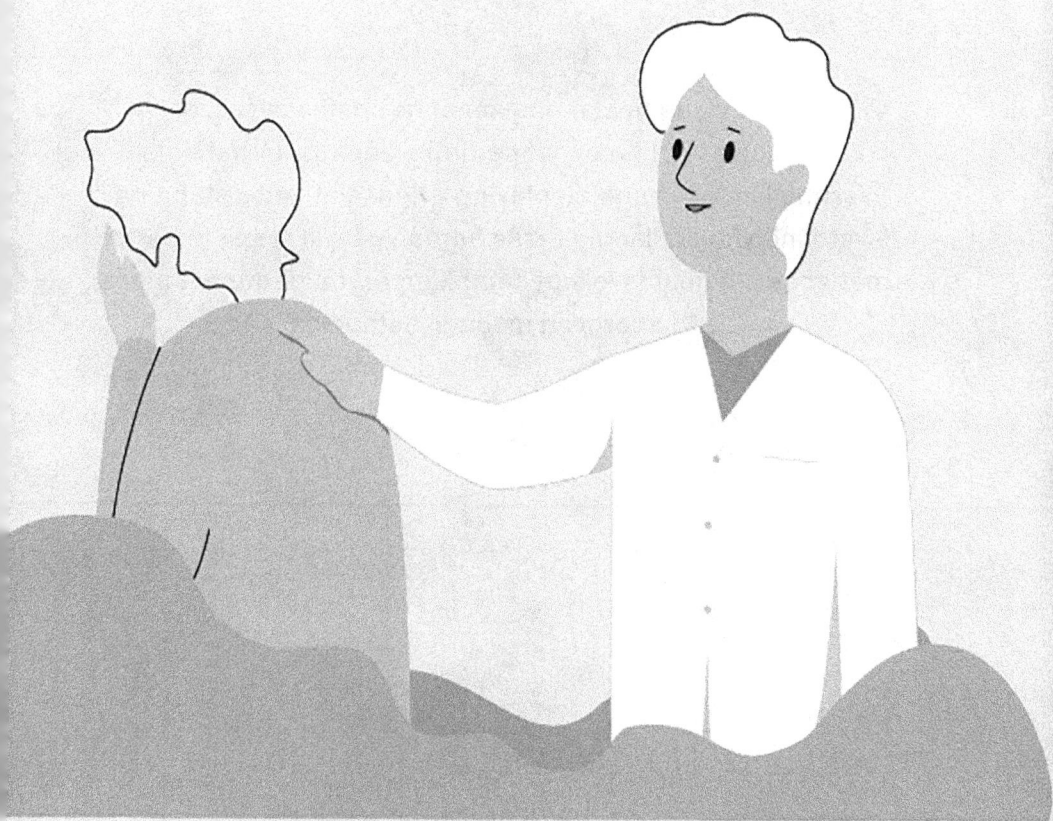

To be a good healer, one must be compassionate.
This involves acting on empathetic feelings for patients.
Exerting kindness and displaying a sense of understanding
toward individuals facing these hardships will result in better
experiences, higher levels of compliance with treatment plans,
and improved medical outcomes.

Chapter 8

My Story

"America's healthcare system is in crisis precisely because we systematically neglect wellness and prevention."

—**Tom Harkin**

Before we go any further, I wanted to spend some time writing about my own background and how I came to be writing this book. Most of my patients know me as the founder of R3 Health and MEDHOUSE, innovative integrative and regenerative medicine practices devoted to helping our patients live healthier, longer lives through a "whole body" approach to medicine. As I constantly advocate and discuss, we believe that personalized healthcare is the key to optimal and balanced wellness, preventing chronic disease, optimizing quality and functionality of life, and managing, slowing down, and inhibiting aging. The idea behind R3 Health, MEDHOUSE, and the R3 Health Network is to practice medicine and educate our community (both patients and other medical practitioners and personnel) in a way that is truly patient-centric and empowering—and I believe the unusual path I took to operating successful integrative and regenerative medicine practices that has one foot each in the world of traditional medicine and alternative medicine puts me in a unique position to write this book.

I grew up as the son of a New York City fireman. Mine was a hardworking middle-class family, and I was an avid athlete who played multiple sports in high school and two sports at the collegiate level. My involvement in sports gave me a deep interest in the mechanics of the body, and

I was an eager student of both traditional and alternative approaches to peak performance.

In college, when it came time to think about what I wanted to do with my life, I knew I wanted to be in medicine and was very attracted to orthopedics, or the study of joint and bone health. My family, however, didn't have the money to send me to medical school—I had to pay my own way through undergraduate and later graduate school. Knowing that I wanted to be in medicine, without knowing in what exact direction, I explored all the healthcare professions, and weighed the pros versus the cons. The thought of enrolling in medical school was not the most appetizing concept as the financial limitations, timeframe to completion, and ensuing monumental debt I would face were all deterring factors.

Without medical school as an option, I enrolled in a graduate program to become a physician's associate. The role of physician's associate (PA-C) is relatively new in medicine; the first physicians' associates programs were launched in the 1960s as a way for veterans who had served as medics in Vietnam to continue practicing medicine. Back then, the thinking was that these medics—most of whom were not practicing MDs—had earned extraordinary experience and needed a way to continue practicing medicine.

Since then, the field of physician associate has grown tremendously. Today, physician associates require at least a master's degree, and just like MDs, we can specialize in any field of medicine. This was actually a big part of the decision-making process for me. As I considered what field of medicine I would want to practice, I found it challenging to decide on one field. Being an athlete, I was attracted to bones, joints, and muscles, which lent itself to an orthopedic career. But also appetizing was the thought of plastic and reconstructive surgery.

So many choices, how could I decide on just one? I couldn't! That's what naturally attracted me to a career as a physician associate. Enrolling in a MD or DO program only allows for one path, a very focused, one-way path with no turn-arounds or do-overs! As I explored the PA-C career, I happily discovered that we were trained as generalized or all-around specialists, and we also had the freedom to change our scope of practice. This is what I wanted, as my natural passion was to help people optimize everything about their bodies, not to mention that I was always fascinated with so many different parts of the human body. I also liked that we were trained in 90 percent of the same curriculum as an MD but in a third of the timeframe. Perfect! I wanted to gather the most amount of information in the shortest amount of time, so I could actually get out there and do what I've always wanted to do, help the world be better, healthier people.

As a PA-C, I am able to take histories, perform examinations, order lab studies and diagnostic tests, prescribe medications, work in surgery, and design treatment plans. In short, PAs can do almost everything full MDs can do, and, in many practices, we are the ones who have the most direct patient contact of anyone on staff, which was also very attractive to me. PA-Cs get to spend the most time with patients. For me, being from New York and a social butterfly, that's what I wanted. I also loved learning about people, what made them tick, and what they enjoy. I was always a pleaser, so allowing me to spend the most amount of time with people was a way to love what I was doing. We really get to know them, understand their concerns, build a relationship, listen well, and truly make a difference in their lives.

Once I decided that a career as a PA-C was for me, I was fortunate enough to get accepted to one the top-three PA-C schools in the country at the time, Quinnipiac University in Connecticut. During my PA-C training, I was eager to continue with a focus on orthopedics and completed two additional rotations (the PA-C form of residency) in orthopedic surgery.

After I completed my training, I took a job with an orthopedic clinic and had my first real-world contact with the world of medicine as a healthcare provider. It was during this first professional job that I realized medicine was not all it was cracked up to be. I quickly saw the pitfalls of healthcare and the "dark side" of medicine in the United States, and I very swiftly learned and figured out why Americans were so unhealthy. Reality was nothing like what they taught us in medical school.

At this clinic, we regularly saw patients coming in for total hip or knee replacements who weren't great candidates for surgery. I can remember having frequent conversations with the surgeon that this patient or that patient would probably have a bad outcome from the surgery, but we'd go ahead and do it anyway. In one particular case, I remember a patient coming in for a total hip replacement while also suffering from uncontrolled type 2 diabetes, COPD, and atrial fibrillation. We counseled the patient on things they should be working on to get healthier before proceeding with the total joint replacement, but the lead surgeon opted to go ahead with the surgery anyway. Not surprisingly, the results were not optimal. The patient had several major complications, including in the hospital while still in the recovery room. After the surgery, it was a two-year marathon of complications, one after the other, including two additional surgeries to minimize the negative effects of the complications from the initial surgery. Ultimately, the patient needed an above-the-knee amputation on the side that did not even get the hip replacement!

Even then, I remember thinking that if we had just taken three to six months to work with this patient to get healthier first, and get their comorbidities under control, their outcome would have been much better. But who was I? I was a recently graduated PA-C who had only been out in the "real world" of medicine for less than two years, going up against the lead orthopedic surgeon of a thirty-physician group with seven offices and more letters than one can count after his name. I would never ever win any debate with the surgeon about whether or not to operate on a patient. Take it from me, sometimes notorious surgeons and tenured and accredited physicians have no shame in boasting about themselves! Every day, I would have conversations with some of the orthopedic doctors about patients and trying to better our patients by getting them to be healthier and maybe even prevent the need for surgery, but to no avail. I would regularly be scolded by my attending physician, who said things like, "Why do I care about their diabetes? I am not their endocrinologist! We're putting in a fake limb so who cares about the circulation and nerve damage that will arise from the elevated insulin and hemoglobin A1C levels? It's not my problem. They should find another primary care physician, one that actually gives a shit!" After two years of this, my eyes were finally opened to the "dark side" of medicine, as I will forever refer to it!

Once I became fully aware of these problems, I was in a tough spot. During my training and before I could practice medicine, I took the same Hippocratic oath that every doctor takes: "I will prevent disease whenever I can, for prevention is preferable to cure." The oath's intent is clear to everyone who takes it. First, we shall do no harm.

Increasingly, however, I felt like it would be impossible to uphold my oath while practicing under these circumstances. Rather than actually helping our patients, in too many cases, I saw a clinic under financial pressure to perform as many surgeries as possible and push patients through who weren't ready for their procedures. After a short time, I was so fed up that I was ready to make a major shift away from conventional medicine and get into another scope of medicine. But would I be able to find what I was looking for? My dream job? Up until that point, I had no idea that integrative medicine existed because it sure as hell was not presented to us in PA-C training!

At the time, this was a terrifying choice, and success was far from guaranteed, but I knew that if I really wanted to help people, I would have to change the way I was practicing medicine, even if it meant re-learning a lot of things I thought I already knew. Even if it meant taking a new job and moving away from New York, where I grew up, to a new practice in

South Florida. Even if it meant going back for more training in the field of integrative and regenerative medicine, fields I'd learned absolutely nothing about in school. I knew there had to be a better way to practice medicine, there had to be a better way to actually make good on my Hippocratic oath. There had to be a better way to make a difference!

After working in conventional medicine for almost two years, I finally mustered up enough courage to take advantage of my PA training and switch into clinical practice in a brand-new scope of practice: integrative and regenerative medicine. Keep in mind, this leap was forcing me to leave a higher guaranteed salary in the northeast and move to the unknown Wild West of medicine in South Florida, where I was taking a position that involved a lot of self-teaching and additional fellowship (basically going back to school) for a fraction of pay I was earning in a sub-specialty like orthopedics. But the choice was a no-brainer. I could not continue doing what I was doing. It was not even practicing medicine. Most times, I felt as though I was part used-car salesman and part auto mechanic (no disrespect to those professions!).

I had first learned of integrative and regenerative medicine from a patient I saw in my job in orthopedics. I always enjoyed seeing this patient as we talked about natural supplements the patient had been using and reading about. This patient—my "aura patient" as I refer to him—really opened my eyes to a whole new world of medicine I knew very little about but had known since high school that I wanted to work in.

My aura patient thankfully lit the spark that allowed me to take a leap of faith and transition into a new area of medicine, one that was never really spoken about and only discussed behind closed doors and amongst families in secrecy. This area of medicine was ignored by conventional healthcare or derided as "voodoo" medicine. I enrolled in the American Academy of Anti-Aging Medicine (A4M) fellowship program, and it was here my life changed. Here I learned about topics I had only dreamed about, things that were very contrary to my training in medical school but made so much sense to me. After completing this intense, almost two-year fellowship/residency program, I knew I had made the right move to get out of conventional healthcare. It just felt right.

After completing my A4M fellowship training program, I happily took my first job in integrative and regenerative medicine as a director for a large and very successful integrative medicine clinic in South Florida. I was enthralled with this position because it was working right alongside one of the field's most renowned and contributing physicians, Dr. Alfred Sears. In Sears's clinic, I saw an entirely new way of practicing medicine and was introduced to integrative and functional medicine actually being used with patients.

This type of medicine viewed patients as whole people and sought to give them the tools and knowledge they needed to practice good self-care and prevent disease. Like the name implies, integrative medicine takes the full range of human experience into account, paying attention not only to the physical aspects of disease but also the mental, emotional, psychological, and even spiritual aspects of health. For the next three years, my life was a blur of practicing medicine and learning. I was working up to eighty hours a week at the clinic while also completing additional fellowships and advanced regenerative-medicine residencies. I soon became a nationally recognized physician trainer in advanced regenerative modalities, techniques such as PRP, stem cell therapy, peptides, and functional medicine. Not only was I treating and educating patients, I was also training doctors from around the world in the amazing field of integrative and regenerative medicine.

The only word for this period is "intense." I actually felt like I was back in PA-C school, where it was common practice to be in didactic lecture for twelve hours then in a physiology lab for four hours, only to go home and study for another four hours! To quote my PA-C program director, it was like "trying to drink out of a firehose"! But I didn't care. I loved every minute of what I was doing. My interactions with patients were detailed; I had time to listen and understand their problems. I had time to develop treatment plans. This was the medicine I had always dreamed of practicing.

At the same time, I was learning about a better way to practice medicine, I was introduced to the business side of medicine—and this was eye-opening. The clinic I worked for was one of the biggest names in the field of alternative medicine, with a high-profile, national reputation. When I first started working there, the clinic physician was involved in patient care, and as director I had the privilege of working personally with every patient who came into the clinic.

Over time, however, I started to notice a change in the way the clinic operated. Our profile was continuing to rise in the alternative medical community, and increasingly I saw profit pressure begin to win out over practicing good medicine. The clinic had introduced a line of supplements and books, and the focus was more and more on supplement sales, which brought in enormous profits with little or no clinical effort. I'll write about this in more depth later, but I was discovering the "dark side" of the alternative medicine movement: profiteering. As I quickly learned, rejecting the framework of conventional medicine doesn't guarantee that healthcare providers are transformed into ethical clinicians with their patients' best interest in mind. Sometimes it just means they want to turn a fast buck.

Once I had this realization, I began to butt heads with the founder of my clinic more frequently. When it became clear that our working relationship couldn't continue, I left that clinic and joined another large anti-aging practice as clinical director—only to once again discover the same thing: a practice driven by profit from supplement sales and recommending procedures that may not be necessary. I tried to make changes at this new clinic, but I ran into stiff resistance.

I was over it, and I had a decision to make. I realized if I wanted to practice medicine the way I wanted to practice medicine—the way that I knew would be best for my patients—I was going to have to take control of my own destiny. I was going to have to open my own clinic. Once again, this was a terrifying and exhilarating thought—running a clinic is a totally different challenge than simply practicing medicine for someone else. There are thousands of administrative issues, from staffing to insurance to the plumbing that I'd have to worry about as an owner versus a staffer. And what did I know about business? Did I earn my MBA from Harvard? Or did I get a medical degree?

Still, by 2016, there was no way around it, and I opened my first clinic. Called RenewU Medical, my new practice leased space from a primary care physician and focused on hormone optimization. My new practice was a whopping 120 square feet (I was renting a room inside the primary care physician's office) that cost $800/month in rent. It was a small start, but I wanted to be careful and see if this new approach would actually work. Not to mention I was still working full-time at the other anti-aging office, while seeing RenewU Medical patients at nights and on the weekends. During this phase of life, there were periods I was working more than a hundred hours per week. Yet although I barely had time to sleep and eat, I was loving life and loving what I was building!

It didn't take long to get my answer. As soon as I started seeing patients on my own at RenewU Medical, many of my old patients followed me. We began to grow, and within a short time, RenewU Medical needed more office space and help and could expand beyond hormone optimization into new therapeutic areas. Our practice was based on the idea that we wanted to create lifelong partnerships with our patients—we wanted to truly work with patients to understand their lifestyle, their health needs and concerns, and create highly personalized care plans that were regularly updated to evolve with how their bodies were evolving. Our unique core philosophy made our practice unique, and our patients' successes were our greatest marketing tool. I had ZERO marketing budget unlike other clinics, but our patients were our best referral source. Every month, patients referred family members and friends, and we continued to grow exponentially. As a result of the growing business, we could charge lower initial consultation fees than most similar clinics and spent time with new and prospective patients to really understand what they needed to remain healthy.

A New Type of Medical Practice

From the very beginning, I knew I wanted to run a different kind of clinic, one that avoided both the pitfalls of conventional medical offices and the issues that too many alternative medical clinics experience. Along the way, I recognized certain signs that a medical practice may not be operating with your health first. Some of these clues include:

- Too many newsletters (or newsletters that have more used-car salesman vibes than educational information), emails, and mailers. Most hospitals and clinics do some marketing—it's an important way to get the word out—but excessive marketing is usually a sign that the clinic is prioritizing profit. No medical clinic needs to send out 100 or 150 emails a month.

- Aggressive sales techniques for supplements. Dietary supplements are an important part of most treatment plans, and it's vital to use high-quality supplements. However, supplements are also the catnip of the medical world—they are easy to formulate and brand and can be highly profitable if people cut corners.

- Very expensive initial consultations. Some of the more well-known "media docs" charge outrageous fees for an initial consultation. The point of this consultation is for patients to get a sense of the clinic and for caregivers to learn more about the patient's unique health needs. This visit is meant to lay the groundwork for a future relationship, not pad the clinic's bottom line. (This is why we do our first consultation for free.)

- Requiring patients to undergo every diagnostic test under the sun before the initial consult. These tests are often paid for directly by the patient, and there's no reason for a healthcare provider to require thousands or tens of thousands of dollars of testing before you meet. That should only come after the initial consultation and any preliminary screening exams, which are usually covered by insurance.

- Dirty, disorganized office and treating spaces. A clinic should operate like a well-oiled, efficient, and organized machine. There should be advanced and current technologies available at every stage of the process, from gathering histories and intake to diagnostic testing and screening. Chaos is not welcome—the space should be calm and elegant, informative, and welcoming.

Even if a clinic does meet all of these criteria, it's still vital that patients are comfortable with their healthcare provider and vibe with him or her. Lost in all of the numbers and statistics is a very real truth: medicine is about people on both sides of the table communicating and interacting about their wellness plan. Your healthcare journey should be two-sided, not a healthcare dictatorship. The practitioner should be learning just as much from you as you learn from the practitioner. Ultimately, patients should know they are respected and their concerns will be taken seriously, that they will have a voice in their own care and they will be heard. These are the principles I founded my practices on, and they've served my patients well—even after most of them have been disillusioned, confused, and even sickened by previous care. We spend a lot of time in our clinics solving problems and educating patients, but when it comes to creating fully empowered patients, there's no such thing as trying too hard.

Today, we continue to have success in our clinics because we are genuine, empathetic, sincere, preach education and awareness to our patients, have built a wellness community and established long-term relationships with our patients, don't pretend to be a used-car salesman, and we genuinely make a difference in our patients' quality of life and continuity of care. We help our patients achieve their short-term and long-term goals by optimizing quality and functionality of life with the goal to ensure vitality and longevity.

Chapter 9

Homeostasis:
The Key to Health

"Dynamic means that whenever a part of the system is out of balance, the rest of the members of the system will try to bring it back into balance."

—John Bradshaw

Now that you know something more about my background, I want to spend a little time exploring the philosophy that drives not only my medical practices but our approach with our patients and my own life. This core philosophy is essential to understanding how to maintain optimal health, prolonged functionality, vitality, and longevity.

One of the reasons I switched gears from practicing in conventional medicine to integrative and regenerative medicine was my thorough fascination with the complexity of the human body, including the billions of physiological chemical reactions that happened in the few seconds it took you to read that last sentence. We all are familiar with the miracle of childbirth and the process of growing an unfertilized egg into an embryo and then into a human with lungs developed enough to born and breath air—but how much do we know about what happens after that baby is born? The average man and woman now lives to seventy and seventy-two years old, respectively. With what you know goes on in the womb in nine months, imagine what happens in the remaining seventy-plus years of life! Think about that for a minute and you'll understand why I am so fascinated with the human body and how it works. This concept further solidifies why I decided to live my life and help and educate other people on these critical concepts.

It's important for us as individuals to recognize and appreciate the complexity and dynamic nature of the human body. Simply put, the human body is an extraordinary development, with many complex systems running alongside each other to support physiologic functionality. Our major organ systems—cardiovascular, pulmonary, orthopedic, neurologic, gastrointestinal, etc.—are designed to carry out specific functions that allow us to move, communicate, laugh, love, explore the sensory world, and even determine right from wrong. In optimal health, all these systems work together in a coordinated web to confer energy, resistance to disease, and vibrant activity. During these periods—which includes the effortless health of youth for many people—all of the body's systems are balanced in support of one another. This condition is called *homeostasis*, which is defined by Oxford as "the tendency toward a relatively stable equilibrium between interdependent elements." Another definition I like from the medical textbook Mosby is: "A property of cells, tissues, organelles, and organisms that allows the maintenance and regulation of the stability needed to function properly. Homeostasis is a healthy state that is maintained by the constant adjustment of biochemical and physiological pathways."

Simply put, homeostasis is our bodies' system of checks and balances. The process of homeostasis allows for our different organ systems to interact and balance each other. There is a wonderful example I frequently use to explain this concept to our patients. When we breathe in air while having a lung disease such as chronic obstructive pulmonary disease (COPD) or emphysema, our body cannot regulate its alkalinity levels (pH levels), including oxygen and carbon dioxide (CO_2) balance, correctly. This affects our overall acidity or alkalinity. If your lungs are not working properly, not allowing for the expelling of CO_2 on their own, then your body can become too acidic (lower pH levels). We call this respiratory acidosis. As your body retains CO_2, it lingers in the bloodstream and instead of transporting freshly oxygenated blood to all your vital organs, you start to transport acidic CO_2 to all your organs, which is why respiratory acidosis is a potentially lethal complication. In turn, respiratory acidosis causes your kidneys (one of your body's other filter systems) to initiate their own checks and balances, which changes the way your kidneys resorb certain alkaline compounds such as sodium bicarbonate to help balance out the acidity and make the body more alkaline (higher pH levels). You can see how dysfunction in one system—the lungs—cascades into problems in another, the kidneys. This interdependence happens thousands of times throughout the body.

Disease occurs when one or more of these systems falls out of balance, or when homeostasis breaks down, the most obvious manifestation of dysfunction. Heart disease, diabetes, arthritis, Alzheimer's disease, and even cancer are all signs that homeostasis has not only broken down but has been breaking down for a long time. In an optimally functioning body, many of the underlying disease processes that drive these dreaded conditions are corrected and managed automatically, thus reducing the risk of actually developing the disease. Over time, however, as the body ages, the fragile biological machinery often inhibits homeostasis, resulting in a cascade of downstream effects that encourage disease, just as we saw in the earlier example of lung disease. Without proper attention and care, it's only a matter of time until full-blown diseases develop, and by the time that happens, the damage has been done and it's much harder to correct the underlying conditions that caused it.

In fact, the presence of disease is actually the last step in the breakdown of homeostasis. The breakdown of homeostasis usually happens long before any symptoms are noticeable, often years before. It begins at the cellular level, as the subtle processes that keep your body healthy are sabotaged and assaulted by disease-causing agents including toxins from the environment, unhealthy food, or microorganisms like viruses, fungi, and bacteria. At first, the body might easily fend off these attacks, but after years of working to protect itself, the body's defenses are worn down and the disease process can begin in earnest. This is one of the most critical components for people to understand about how our bodies not only work but age. Remember, one small imbalance to this system of homeostasis does not affect only that one part of the process; instead, one small impurity or non-efficiency rapidly cascades into affecting many other organ systems. This is why it is nonsensical that we have so many practicing sub-sub-specialists out there. If a sub-specialist only focuses on their one sub-specialty area, they fail to recognize where the problem started and/or what other areas the lack of homeostasis is affecting. This is why, as an individual, if you see all these sub-specialists it can be very difficult to feel well. They fail to look at the body as a whole or, even worse—fail to communicate with each other in an attempt to get your body working as a whole!

Inflammation: Enemy of Homeostasis

One of the best indicators that homeostasis is threatened or the process has started to degrade is the presence of inflammation throughout the body. In recent years, we've begun to get a much clearer understanding of how destructive chronic inflammation is to your cells and tissues. This type of chronic inflammation is distinguished from the immediate swelling we experience after an injury, which is known as acute inflammation. Acute inflammation is designed by nature to help our bodies heal and actually is a way of protecting our bodies from further injury or damage. Inflammation in an acute setting is a series of events that our bodies kick into gear when there is an acute injury, active disease, or foreign intruder. Depending on the site of injury and the mechanism of injury, inflammation presents itself with the five characteristics most of us are familiar with: pain, redness, immobility, swelling, and heat.

Chronic inflammation is more like a slow-burning fire raging throughout the body, as dangerous pro-inflammatory chemicals mount a relentless siege on healthy cells, eventually triggering an immune-system reaction that makes things worse. In fact, this type of long-term inflammation is the underlying cause of a huge number of diseases that Americans suffer from today, including the deadliest disease in the country and the leading killer of both men and women: heart disease. It's well established now that by the time most people suffer a heart attack or acute coronary event, there is almost always a long history of atherosclerosis, or hardening of the arteries, that contributed to that event. And the underlying cause of atherosclerosis? Inflammation in the artery wall.

This process has been studied extensively since it was first proposed in the 1990s. Today, we understand that atherosclerosis begins in the thin, delicate inner layers of the coronary arteries, or endothelium. In a normal situation, these cells are smooth and resistant to injury or blood clots. If the endothelium is damaged, however, tiny tears in the endothelial layer attract immune system cells, which adhere to the artery wall and form a thin plaque. The most common causes of injury to the endothelial cells include an unhealthy diet high in saturated fat, smoking, lack of exercise, and high levels of toxins. Once a plaque has formed, an inflammation cascade begins whereby immune system cells penetrate into the artery wall further, which stimulates an even stronger immune system response. Before long, the combination of lipids in the artery wall, immune system factors, and pro-inflammatory chemicals forms a larger plaque that is protected by a hard, fatty plaque covering. This covering, in turn, attracts calcium, which adheres to the growing plaque and causes the artery to lose its supple elasticity. Thus the blood vessel become rigid and loses its ability to contract and pump blood, and it also impedes blood to freely flow through, a double whammy.

At this point, the atherosclerotic process is well underway, as the plaque continues to excrete pro-inflammatory chemicals, attract calcium, oxidize fatty acids, and get bigger. If the plaque eventually gets big enough and remains unstable, it can rupture, sending bits of plaque downstream to block smaller arteries, while also causing a blood clot to form at the site of the rupture.* This is known as a heart attack. And as scary as all that sounds, what makes that scenario worse is that most of the time this process happens slowly over years, without you even knowing it or feeling any of these changes!

The heart isn't alone when it comes to the dangers of rampant inflammation. Diseases as diverse as arthritis, allergies, celiac disease, inflammatory bowel disorders, diverticulitis and many others are all caused by long-term, chronic inflammation.† In each case, an inflammatory response is triggered that sets off a cascade of intensifying reactions that contribute to a worsened disease state.

We need to help people understand the concept of inflammation at the cellular and physiologic level. It is at the cellular level that inflammation really destroys our body's functionality and physiology and impedes healing, decreasing functionality and shortening longevity. This is why inflammation should really be deemed "the silent killer" rather than high blood pressure. When inflammation starts at the cellular level, our bodies can employ many compensation mechanisms that can adapt, but over time these episodes of inflammation create problems of monstruous proportions by disrupting the normal cell function and bringing the body to a state from which it is much harder to improve.

When a cell is not working like it's supposed to, it is programmed to recognize the dysfunction and start a process called apoptosis or programmed cell death. Instead of the cell not working well and creating more inflammation, it is programmed to self-destruct, so it won't negatively influence other cells or go through a mutation (change in DNA) and become pre-cancerous or cancerous. The problem is when enough of these

---

* Danesh J, Wheeler JG, Hirschfield GM, Eda S, Eiriksdottir G, Rumley A, Lowe GD, Pepys MB, -- V. C-reactive protein and other circulating markers of inflammation in the prediction of coronary heart disease. *N J Med.* 2004 Apr 1;350(14):1387-97.
† Wikipedia. Inflammation. https://en.wikipedia.org/wiki/Inflammation#Inflammatory_disorders.

cells die, it causes specific glandular and organ disease, as well as cancer stem cell stimulation. Alternatively, enough of one specific cell type dying off does not allow for that tissue to work sufficiently. In fact, the most worrisome medical condition you've probably never heard about is something called *systemic chronic inflammation (SCI).**

Diseases of inflammation cannot be "cured" by looking at the disease and trying to cure it. Rather, we need to focus on the environment that influences the inflammation and allows the disease to develop. Remember, when a disease finally presents itself, it is after a longer, tedious process of subtle change and loss of homeostasis. This is why integrative medicine looks at early indicators of the disease process, things your normal PCP may not even know about like homocysteine, CRP-HS, cortisol, and other blood markers. These laboratory values are the earliest and most critical detectors of inflammation and premature aging. We need to better understand the inflammation that is happening throughout the body and try to be as proactive as we can to identify, evaluate, and inhibit the process of inflammation because no matter what our genetic pre-disposition is or how clean our lifestyles are, our bodies will produce inflammation.

To make it worse, unfortunately many of the things we accept as "normal" in modern life are highly inflammatory, including foods and drinks that millions of people take into their bodies every day. This includes everything from the dangerous trans fats that are used to keep baked goods "shelf stable" for months at time to the ubiquitous alcohol consumption that drenches society. Besides diet, other factors that promote runaway inflammation include lack of exercise, smoking, and living in a highly polluted area. A young person who eats an unhealthy diet, gets no exercise, and drinks alcohol might look healthy on the outside, but it's likely that his or her cells are already under sustained assault from pro-inflammatory chemicals, setting the course for future disease. And we must recognize that even one minor contributor to inflammation can initiate the process of loss of homeostasis and cellular inflammation. So, eating healthy is not a justification for consuming too much alcohol, not getting enough exercise, or compensating for living in a highly polluted city! Remember, the body is the sum of all its parts!

As grim as this sounds—surrounded on all sides by foods and conditions that promote inflammation and encourage disease—there is good news in this research. Because we've identified inflammation as a key destabilizer of homeostasis, it means we have a roadmap to preventing

---

* https://www.nature.com/articles/s41591-019-0675-0.

disease over the long term: reduce inflammation. This typically begins with a full work-up, including blood work, to measure inflammatory blood markers and get an idea of the inflammatory burden any particular person is carrying.

Once we've created a detailed picture of a patient's full health status based on their blood markers and a detailed history, we can begin to create a treatment plan and start the process of inhibiting inflammation and reducing the inflammatory burden on our bodies. In fact, the most important thing anyone can do to reduce their inflammatory risk is to get educated. For some people, this is not an elaborate process, but it is perhaps the first and most important stepping-stone to improving our health. Knowledge—how to eat well, how to live a healthy lifestyle with plenty of exercise and not smoking—is the best prescription. This is a message that's knitted deeply into everything I do as a healthcare provider and the core foundation of how our clinics operate. First, we create a thorough picture of a person's underlying health, and then we provide information on concrete steps they can take to improve their health.

While this type of medicine is within the reach of any healthcare professional, there are powerful forces working against most physicians even if they understand the underlying concept. For this approach to work, a few conditions must be in place:

1. The healthcare provider needs to establish a long-term relationship with that patient. In a world of largely disposable relationships, it can't be stressed enough how important an enduring provider/patient relationship can be. People change over time— the healthcare needs of a patient at twenty will be dramatically different than the needs of that same patient at forty, sixty, or eighty. While it might be too much to ask that patients stick with their same practitioner for decades, it is critical to recognize that patients have ever-evolving medical needs. There is no cookie-cutter approach to medicine that works.

2. Patients need to have a complete understanding of what's going on and what they can do to maintain health. The old top-down "doctor knows best" paradigm isn't enough to get people to make positive, permanent changes in their behavior. Not only do practitioners not have adequate time to educate properly, but patients will only make those types of changes if they really understand why it makes sense to skip that fast-food hamburger

or cut down on their drinking—it takes a lot to overcome the pull of immediate gratification and cultural pressure.

3. Providers need to have the time to attend to every patient as a whole person. This doesn't just mean time in the patient room, although that's important. As a healthcare provider, it's almost impossible to really assess someone's health in a rushed five-minute office visit, so it does matter that the provider has plenty of time to spend with patients during routine well-visits. More than that, however, it's also important that patients are routinely followed. For many people, especially older people, a fifteen-minute well-check every six months, including a handful of basic blood tests, is just woefully inadequate to understand their true health condition. In reality, blood testing should be conducted every few months to establish baselines and identify trends, and patients should be closely monitored to make sure their goals are being met.

The idea here is to gain a complete understanding of a person's health, especially what's going on internally, and craft a care plan that supports their short- and long-term health and inhibits or slows inflammation while maintaining homeostasis. This may mean prescribing supplements to address a nutrient deficiency, or using bioidentical hormones to correct an imbalance, or recommending lifestyle changes in conjunction with peptides that can help reduce damaging cholesterol or help control elevated glucose levels. We want to be proactive instead of reactive, but if someone has been under the influence of these inflammatory and homeostatic changes, there are wonderful, natural, and regenerative approaches to help reverse the damage.

Ideally, customized treatment plans should support anabolism and discourage catabolism. Anabolism is known as the "building state," where the body uses energy to create large molecules that are used to support healthy function. In contrast, catabolism is the state in which the body breaks down large molecules to release energy, such as breaking the stored form of glucose, glycogen, into glucose molecules for energy consumption.* Although these concepts are widely used in exercise—here "anabolic" exercises are ones like weight lifting that build muscle while "catabolic" exercises are

---

* BYJU'S. Differences between catabolism and anabolism. https://byjus.com/biology/differences-between-catabolism-and-anabolism/.

ones like running that use energy—these are actually metabolic processes that are regulated by sex hormones like estrogen and testosterone, as well as cortisol and adrenaline. An anabolic state means that the body's endocrine system is supporting healthy function and muscle development, an increasingly important part of health and longevity as people age.

Alternative Versus Traditional: A False Dichotomy

These are the broad outlines and some of my core philosophies, and it's important that healthcare providers use all the tools available to them to help their patients. It's unfortunate that so much of the medical world has divided itself into two opposing camps: traditional medicine versus so-called alternative medicine. This false dichotomy has the effect of discrediting viable therapies from both "sides." For some people, any type of pharmaceutical is viewed with suspicion and hostility, as if all prescription drugs are part of a plot by pharmaceutical companies. For others, alternative medicine is largely viewed as a get-rich-quick scam run by unscrupulous doctors and supplement companies who prey on people's ignorance. And that is no exaggeration—there are times where this emotion persists amongst patients, practitioners, and the medical community.

In fact, the goal of all healthcare providers should be to use any approach that works—while simultaneously working to understand how a particular treatment will work with a patient's unique biology and lifestyle. This point is essential: all of us are biologically different, so what works for one person may not work as well for someone else. This is why it's essential that patients receive regular, personal attention and monitoring, so care plans can be adjusted.

In my practices, we are open to anything that works, no matter which side of the alternative versus traditional medicine divide it comes from. Yes, this does mean that we have to spend valuable time staying up to date with current research, going far beyond the reference ranges that are treated like received wisdom, but this is a crucial part of delivering effective healthcare. Remember: the practice of bloodletting was accepted as cutting-edge medicine for two thousand years and has only been abandoned relatively recently.

With this in mind, here are a few of the treatment modalities we use in our clinics. My goal here isn't to convince you that any particular treatment is superior to another, but to show the breadth of tools we have available to support lasting health, ensuring homeostasis, inhibiting inflammation, improving longevity, and enhancing quality of life.

Hormone Optimization. Hormone status is one of the most important indicators of health. As young people, our endocrine systems are typically balanced and designed to support vibrant health and disease protection. As we age, however, hormone production gradually changes and in some cases, ceases. As women age, their production of estrogen and progesterone drops dramatically. The result is increased risk of heart attack (heart disease is the leading killer of women) and osteoporosis, as well as the symptoms of menopause including hot flashes, vaginal dryness, and mood changes. For men, the decline in hormone status isn't as abrupt, but it's no less dramatic. Known as andropause, testosterone production in men begins to decline about 1.5 percent per year around age thirty-five. By age seventy, a typical man is producing a fraction as much testosterone as he did in his thirties, resulting in decreased muscle mass and muscle wasting, increased risk of osteoporosis, erectile dysfunction, and mood changes.

As you can see, both men and women have very complicated and complex hormone profiles, all of which fluctuate, interact, and influence each other. If even one hormone starts to become imbalanced, it can affect every hormone in the endocrine system. This applies to all hormones, not just sex hormones. Thyroid and adrenal hormones are just as important to the aging process, and these too often are overlooked, underappreciated, and ignored. Hormone therapy is the practice of carefully measuring hormone levels, then implementing treatment programs to achieve hormonal balance and optimization.

Nutraceuticals. Once again, aging has a profound effect on the body's ability to use or manufacture essential nutrients. As we get older and our gut microbiome changes, as well as our basic cell efficiency and even our diet, it becomes harder and harder for our bodies to efficiently extract nutrients from the food we eat. At the same time, our modern food supply and diets are already wildly deficient in many essential nutrients, leading to widespread nutrient deficiencies even among young people. Among older people, deficiencies of vitamin B12, calcium, iron, and magnesium are common. The solution here is to get an accurate picture of the patient's overall health status and then prescribe supplementation to restore adequate blood levels of vital nutrients. This may be accomplished through regular supplementation, or through IV therapy in the clinic.

Platelet-Rich Plasma (PRP) Therapy. PRP therapy is a well-validated approach to muscular, joint, soft tissue, facial, and hair injury. In this approach, patients are treated with their own plasma in which blood platelets are super concentrated. As it turns out, platelets (which cause blood to clot and stop a cut from bleeding) contain and release thousands of substances called cytokines and chemokines, which have thousands of effects in our body, including anti-inflammatory, building tissue, creating amino acids, and stimulating the immune system, stem cells, and more. PRP injections trigger the patient's own immune system and healing functions to help repair torn tissues or injuries like torn Achilles' tendons or rotator cuffs. This approach has been shown to reduce pain and improve healing times.*

Stem Cell Therapy. Stem cell therapy is another relatively new modality that relies on injections of activated stem cells to help repair and replenish damaged cells. Stem cells are primitive cells that haven't yet specialized into different types of cells. Injecting stem cells has been a standard part of leukemia treatment for years—patients are injected with stem cells to replace cancerous bone marrow cells that have been killed by radiation therapy. Outside of cancer treatment, stem cell therapy can be used to target various medical conditions to help restore and regenerate damaged organs, bones, and tissues without surgery. Stem cells can come from donor tissues, or we can harvest your own de-activated stem cells and reactivate them so they can function how they did in your younger years. Donor stem cells are obtained from birth tissues such as umbilical cord tissue, umbilical cord blood, amniotic tissue, or amniotic fluid.

Stem cell and exosome therapies are some of the most fascinating medical treatments that are helping to improve chronic inflammatory medical conditions that have been resistant to conventional therapies. In our practice, we use stem cell therapy to help improve patients' health in many different ways: orthopedic, kidney, liver, GI, blood disorders, degenerative neurogenic disease, chronic lung disease, and even as preventive means. And yes, it is legal and performed very safely and efficiently.

Peptide Therapies. Peptides are amino acids that work together to control many body functions, from hormone production to the creation of the cellular matrix that provides structure to our tissues and organs. Similar to nutrients and hormones, as we age our production of peptides decreases, and our ability to use peptides also declines. The result is a peptide deficiency that increases your risk of disease and cellular breakdown. Peptide therapies are designed to identify which peptides are in decline and replenish their supply. This is commonly used to improve skin conditions, as well as improve autoimmune disorders and hormone imbalance.

---

* Hospital for Special Surgery, New York City. Platelet-rich plasma. https://www.hss.edu/condition-list_prp-injections.asp.

Intravenous Therapies (IV): I'm not just talking about IV fluids or the "hangover" clinics you may have seen trending in the last few years. In fact, this is likely one of integrative and regenerative medicine's most scrutinized and abused treatment modalities. In reality, IV therapies are where we are able to not only identify and replenish key essential micronutrients, coenzymes, and anti-inflammatory substances, but these treatments also allow us to deliver key anti-aging and regenerative substances like ozone (O3) and nicotinamide adenine dinucleotide, better known as NAD, which aid the body in too many ways to list but most importantly stimulate the immune system; have incredible antibacterial, anti-viral, and anti-parasitic effects; and significantly enhance mitochondrial efficiency and longevity.

This list is far from complete but is meant to give you an idea of the tools innovative healthcare providers can use to help patients renew and regenerate at the cellular level. Combined with careful attention to a patient's unique health status and needs, a comprehensive program can be designed that will not only reduce the risk of disease or lessen the effects of an existing condition but actually help the body to restore more youthful function. The results can be overwhelming for individuals—we see and hear this every day, with patients reporting feeling better, having more energy and improved libido, experiencing less pain and symptoms from chronic conditions, and even discontinuing pharmaceuticals.

As a final note, it's important to emphasize the role of patient education. If the goal is to create fully autonomous patients, it's essential that patients have at least a basic understanding of these sometimes-complex therapies and how they work together. It's equally important they understand their own role in their care plan. These are two core philosophies of mine: educating our patients on all aspects of medicine and giving patients the tools they need to make their own healthcare decisions and be their own health advocate.

Lifestyle factors—the medical industry's somewhat dry term for healthy living—remain by far the most important step for most people to maintain health as they age. Patients who understand the value of eating well, getting enough exercise, reducing stress, and getting enough sleep are more likely to take active steps to safeguard their own health, which, in turn, will support whatever therapies they are on. For these patients, knowledge, targeted therapies, and a close partnership with their healthcare provider becomes a virtuous circle that restores homeostasis, inhibits inflammation, and promotes years of improved quality of life and reduced disease risk—and isn't the goal for everyone?

Chapter 10

A Better
Healthcare System

"*The bottom line: Healthcare reform is about the patient, not about the physician.*"

—Abraham Verghese

By now, it should be obvious that I am not one of those people who believe the entire healthcare system should be torn down. In this country, there are certain components of medicine we do well, including trauma, trauma surgery, urgent stabilization, and some surgical specialties. I don't want to naively sit here and say that someone with stage-four pancreatic cancer should not be seeking conventional medical therapies including chemo, radiation, surgery, and medications. That would just be nonsensical.

The key here lies in understanding that there needs to be a more hybrid model, where Eastern and Western medical methodologies can symbiotically combine to yield the best outcomes for those who need more Eastern medicine with supportive Western medicine or vice versa. In many circumstances, there are indications for both in the same scenario.

The system is the product of the sum of its parts, so a poor system is a reflection of poor parts. Throughout this book, I have highlighted some of the critical parts of the system that are set up for failure.

The ultimate goal is to combine what we're doing right with new ideas and new approaches to make sure healthcare truly works for the patients it serves, instead of the large corporate and commercial interests that currently dominate healthcare policy. I believe this revolution can only come from the bottom up—the financial interests in the healthcare industry are far too entrenched to voluntarily give up any of their money or power, even when they come at the expense of patients. Instead, it will require that patients first learn there are better alternatives and then demand change.

I have worked with tens of thousands of patients in both a conventional healthcare setting and an integrative medicine setting. I'm also a healthcare student educator and integrative medicine practitioner trainer. This perspective has allowed me to see firsthand the pitfalls of our current system's successes, accomplishments, challenges, and failures. In this chapter, I hope to express my opinion on how to amend and improve a battered, challenged, and failing system.

My suggested approaches are knitted together by one common idea: that we should be working much harder to prevent disease in the first place rather than waiting for symptoms to emerge and then rushing to treat an already advanced disease process. This is hardly a revolutionary position—almost all of my colleagues would agree that disease prevention is a much better strategy for patients than waiting to treat an existing disease. The disconnect, however, is the willingness to take the steps we need to take to get from here to there. So, what will be the catalyst? How will we get from here to there?

We must educate. Not just educate our patients, practitioners, or students, or governing organizations—we must EDUCATE EVERYONE! The approaches I'll discuss in this chapter all represent pieces of the same puzzle, but I firmly believe this kind of change is possible. We *can* change the way our healthcare providers think and process information. We can change the process so practitioners actually have time to take in and use information. We need to change how healthcare providers communicate with patients, how healthcare practitioners communicate with each other, how healthcare providers communicate with other medical personnel, and how healthcare providers communicate with those who operate the business of medicine. It is only when we do these things—and do *all* of these things—that we'll be able to really improve our healthcare system. So, with that said, let's explore the concepts and therapies that I have been using in my medical practice over the last ten years with great success.

Functional Medicine

Functional medicine is a relatively new approach to practicing medicine. According to the Institute for Functional Medicine, this approach "determines how and why illness occurs and restores health by addressing the root cause of disease for each individual."*

Functional medicine practitioners take the time to fully understand their patients, their health, and the lifestyle factors that may be influencing the development of a disease, then create unique, customized care plans for each patient. The goal is to encourage patients to take steps to prevent disease based on each patient's unique needs. This means the healthcare provider needs a detailed understanding of that patient's full history to aid in actually determining the root causes of disease, including their family history, lifestyle factors, genetic factors that may put them at risk for certain conditions, hormone status, nutrient status, and even mental health status. Health is a choice and not a fate; we know that the choices we make and the way we live our lives actually impact our health more than our genetics. In short, in functional medicine, anything that can affect the patient's disease risk is critical information to help a practitioner understand their patient and what etiology their conditions are stemming from—whether it's a family history of heart attack or elevated inflammatory markers in their blood.

A good way to think of this is by picturing an iceberg. It's a well-known fact that the visible part of the iceberg represents only a fraction of the iceberg's total size. The rest is submerged. This is where the saying, "That's only the tip of the iceberg" comes from: only the tip is really visible, while the bulk of the iceberg is hidden below the waves.

Disease and the disease process is a cellular process, and usually by the time a disease is noticed by you or the patient, it's already too late and the disease process has been going on beneath the surface. The actual symptoms are usually just the tip of the iceberg, while the majority of the disease process is happening invisibly at the cellular level. In fact, a single underlying health problem like inflammation can be the root cause of multiple health problems, or conversely, a single health problem might have multiple underlying causes.† Our job as healthcare providers is to look at the whole iceberg so we can address the underlying causes, which will have a ripple effect into disease progression and symptoms.

---

* The Institute for Functional Medicine. Functional medicine. https://www.ifm.org/functional-medicine/.
† The Institute for Functional Medicine. Functional medicine. https://www.ifm.org/functional-medicine/.

Functional medicine emphasizes major components of how our bodies work, including diet, nutrition, vitamins, minerals, amino acids, antioxidant levels, hormone status, thyroid status, and adrenal status, to name a few. Sound foreign? Do you recognize or remember having any of these things looked at or discussed the last time you had blood tests? Chances are they weren't, which is the problem! Going back to our iceberg analogy, in order to understand that iceberg, there needs to be people on land, in the air, and even under to assess the whole thing! It's no different with our bodies. Healthcare practitioners need to be looking at your body from a plethora of angles in order to really assess, understand, and compute what's going on. Unfortunately, chances are good that your health care practitioners are not only omitting these things, or don't know how to check for or interpret these essential measures, but they also don't care!

Functional medicine recognizes how our life choices and lifestyle factors influence our health. Functional medicine practitioners take all of this data into account to ensure we understand the complexities of each patient's body and chemistry based on their lifestyle. In functional medicine, we always preach a whole-body approach, making sure we connect the dots between the different organ systems and understand the root causes of the diseases our patients struggle with. As the name indicates, functional medicine practitioners aim their attention at improving patients' functionality, regardless of how diagnostics may influence our interpretation.

This is a very important concept to understand. One of the main goals of our practice is to help people live their best quality of life for the longest period of time. This goal often gets lost or is unappreciated by conventionally practicing practitioners. In conventional medicine, one of the bigger priorities and goals for any practitioner is making a diagnosis and conducting every test under the sun until a diagnosis is found. The reasoning for this is once there is a diagnosis, the doctor can go to that diagnosis's 'flowchart' and use all the conventional means to treat the diagnosis based on whatever drug or surgery the flowchart dictates. In this approach, there is entirely too much emphasis placed on one condition, one part of the body and more "standardized" process of treatment. Conventionally trained practitioners make all their decisions based on what they see on a scan, or what the blood tests show, versus a functional medicine practitioner who uses data from the diagnostic piece and combines it with all the other data to reach a conclusion.

Have you or anyone you know ever gone for a test or scan or any type of diagnostic work-up and come back with some "incidental finding." This

---

A Dietician's Take on Functional Medicine

Elyse Marrone is the clinical director of the Lifestyle Nutrition Institute in North Palm Beach and a highly sought-after registered dietician and consultant. Elyse is trained in integrated functional medicine and works with dozens of traditional doctors—but it almost didn't happen. She started her career in the hospitals in the 1990s, when "dieticians" were not respected. At one point, she remembers a doctor questioning why she was bothering with patient recommendations at all, saying, "What you do is so boring and won't make any difference. Why do it?"

But today, she is a firm believer in the power of integrated, functional medicine. "In a functional medicine clinic, they do a full assessment of the patient's whole history and make recommendations." For Elyse, this usually includes a recommendation to focus on whole foods and high-quality supplements while cutting out fad diets and inflammatory foods.

---

means they were looking for something completely different but happened to discover this other thing. In many cases, that incidental finding sends you on a wild goose chase to find a diagnosis so it can be treated. This happens all too often in conventional medicine, and that is because conventional medicine places all of its emphasis on diagnostic data!

The good news is that it is possible to bring the concepts associated with functional medicine forward even in a traditional, insurance-based clinical practice. It's true there are challenges associated with convincing insurers to cover the extra level of care required by functional medicine, including more comprehensive diagnostic testing, but as more patients learn about and demand this type of care, I expect insurance companies will respond with policies that make it easier to incorporate functional medicine into any practice.

Integrative Medicine

Integrative medicine is another common approach that attempts to fix many of the issues with our current healthcare system. Broadly speaking, integrative medicine takes into account all of the patient's factors that might be affecting their health, casting a wider net than even functional medicine. This includes emotional and mental health, spirituality and faith, and the strength of patients' social connections.

Importantly, integrative medicine has gone further than older schools of thought in integrating so-called alternative medical modalities with traditional allopathic medicine. Practitioners are taught not only to use prescription medications and surgeries, but also to evaluate alternative approaches and incorporate high-quality alternative treatments into their practice. Patients may be prescribed medication, but they may also leave the office with a prescription for therapeutic massage, yoga, or acupuncture, along with supplement recommendations and hormone therapy to correct hormone imbalances.

Integrative medicine is a hybrid medical model with emphasis on more natural and regenerative medicine therapies. Just as in functional medicine, practitioners in this field also aim to ensure longevity through functional aging and ensuring the highest quality of life for the longest period of time. Integrative medicine practitioners often tend to follow medical management similar to primary care practitioners, but from a more natural, regenerative approach that connects the dots between different organ systems. This is where integrative medicine practitioners overcome many of the failures of conventional primary healthcare practitioners: there is no need to go to other sub-specialists. By its nature, integrative medicine alleviates the need to see many specialists.

Patient education is a crucial element of integrative medicine—this approach is only successful when patients are empowered to understand their body's physiologies and be a part of their health journey and make their own health decisions. One of the core beliefs of integrative medicine is that we live in a deeply unhealthy society, where we are encouraged to make unhealthy decisions at every turn, thanks to heavy marketing for unhealthy products or simple social pressure to do things that are bad for our health. The integrative medical practitioner makes it a priority to teach patients how to recognize poor decisions, make better ones, and minimize the negative impacts of certain lifestyles and behaviors.

Integrative medicine and functional medicine overlap in some crucial ways. Both are concerned with patients as a whole and addressing the root cause of disease while empowering patients to prevent disease by making better choices. The main difference lies in the approach to disease—functional medicine encourages both healthcare providers and patients to dig into the root cause of disease and attempts to address those cases with a customized and individualized care plan. Integrative medicine also feels the same way but recognizes there may be short-term reasons to blend in some conventional medical modalities for the shortest period of time possible while working to get back to more natural or functional solutions.

Regenerative Medicine

While functional medicine and integrative medicine are different ways to approach medicine, regenerative medicine can be thought of as a truly new branch of medicine. Regenerative medicine is built on the idea that the body is so amazingly complex that if we support our bodies or put our bodies in the right environment, the body can rebuild and repair itself, or regenerate itself.

Core to this approach is the recognition that the human body changes and evolves over time, and with age, it no longer functions as well as it did in its youth. Even among people who have been careful their whole lives, aging inevitably brings on changes that affect our underlying health. The immune system no longer functions as well as it did. Bones lose their strength and become brittle. Healing time slows down. Our stem cells slow down and turn themselves off. Arteries lose their supple and elastic character and become vulnerable to injury and insult. Our cells no longer replicate as quickly as they once did, and DNA errors accumulate within cells, sometimes giving rise to cancer. Even the senses of taste and smell break down. Not surprisingly, many of these changes are encouraged by underlying chronic inflammation, which hastens decline and encourages the disease process to start and continue to progress.

Regenerative medicine seeks to identify how aging affects our biology and then understand what we can do to slow it down, inhibit it, and, in the case of disease, reverse underlying processes that are making us sick. This often involves designing care protocols that support healthy DNA division, a balanced gut microbiome with plenty of beneficial bacteria to encourage healthy digestion and nutrient absorption, and reduce inflammation throughout the body.

Unlike regular allopathic medicine, regenerative medicine has a strong focus on the cellular and molecular processes that define aging. In fact, the field itself arose from transplant techniques and cell therapies like bone marrow transplants for leukemia patients. From these beginnings, researchers began to experiment with tissue engineering techniques that make it possible to grow new heart valves, for example. At the same time, the study of stem cell therapies really took off. A few examples of regenerative medicine at work include:

1. Stem cell therapy, whereby immature (sometimes referred to as undifferentiated) cells are injected into a patient, where they

mature into specialized, healthy cells that replace damaged or diseased cells. And despite what you have heard, it is legal.

2. Immunomodulation therapy using peptides, ensuring healthy molecules can improve or strengthen the immune system.

3. Regenerative peptides such as BPC-157 (body protective compound). This natural amino acid–based molecule helps the body repair soft and connective tissues, such as ligaments, tendon, cartilage, meniscus, labrum, blood vessels, collagen, and more.

4. Exosome therapy, which uses tiny particles extracted from stem cells to signal stem cells and attract to areas highest in inflammation.

5. Ozone therapy, which delivers a type of specialized oxygen called ozone to provide a higher concentration of oxygen to help in immune modulation, fighting inflammation, and cleansing and detoxification. Ozone therapy also has tremendous anti-cancer and anti-bacterial/viral properties.

While this is one of the more exciting areas of emerging research and clinical practice in medicine, progress has been slowed by ethical considerations (e.g., what role does fetal tissue play in regenerative medicine?). Nevertheless, it's a safe bet we'll continue to see major forward progress in the field of regenerative medicine. I'm particularly passionate about regenerative medicine as I am privileged to train and educate other practitioners around the world in regenerative medicine and have trained over five hundred practitioners from all over the world. One day, we might think nothing of having our own immature stem cells harvested early in life so they can be trained later in a lab setting to literally grow new organs. For now, however, innovative healthcare providers are already using stem cells and other regenerative approaches to reverse or slow aging at a cellular level and treat disease.

Preventive Medicine

Preventive medicine is a medical specialty that focuses on preventing illness, both at the individual and community level. This specialty is recognized by the American Board of Medical Specialties (ABMS). Healthcare providers who want to practice preventive medicine can earn board certification from the American Board of Preventive Medicine (ABPM) by attending an approved training program, then passing a rigorous exam.*

Preventive medicine has three specialty areas: public health and general preventive medicine, occupational medicine, and aerospace medicine. Of these, public health and general preventive medicine focuses on improving the health of the general public and individuals. With a focus on both the individual and the larger community, preventive medicine encourages practices like disease screening, reducing dangerous activities like texting while driving and engaging in risky sex, and finding effective approaches to reduce obesity and encourage healthy practices like eating right and exercising.

While these are common ideas to almost any medical practice, a preventive medicine specialist is trained to work with patients and communities (including businesses and local governments) to bring these tools into widespread practice. As a result of this focus, patient education is once again a critical component of preventive care. Patients who are educated make better decisions about their health, whether it's eating better, asking the right questions, or knowing and understanding ways to help themselves.

At the same time, preventive medicine has a society-wide component that sets it apart. With a stronger focus on public health, one of the goals of preventive medicine is to remove barriers to care. As I've detailed earlier, this is a big task—our medical system is littered with barriers to care. They are financial, cultural, and historical. They range from insurance plans that offer little or no real protection to the relentless focus on cost that is causing many rural hospitals to close. Preventive medical practitioners often work with public health agencies to identify at-risk communities and work to improve their access to healthcare and empower them to act.

Taken together, we can see themes that unite these approaches to medicine. These themes form the backbone of my philosophy as a caregiver:

1. Work to understand the cause of disease

2. Form a real partnership with my patients to understand their needs

3. Create individualized care plans that aim to prevent disease and disability with more frequent communication and monitoring

---

* American Board of Preventive Medicine. The value of certification. https://www.theabpm.org/become-certified/.

4. Give patients the knowledge they need to make healthy decisions so they can preserve their quality of life long into old age—after all, age without good health and quality of life can be miserable for anyone. My goal is to help patients have wonderful quality of life no matter their age and even health status.

Getting It Right

Again, I want to emphasize that I am not 100 percent against conventional medicine—but we need to recognize there is a time and a place where conventional medical means are necessary and a time and a place where there are far more suitable, safer, and more sustainable options. In order to make our healthcare system more effective and improve our health, several things need to happen. We need to educate our practitioners and change the way they are educated and practice medicine. We need to educate patients and consumers on ways they can take control of their health. And we need to challenge the governing institutions and regulating bodies that govern the way medicine is practiced. The financial issues in the current healthcare model are arguably the reason we are in this mess to begin with. However, if we can work with these agencies and insurance companies and transition our business model, real change can happen.

I approach every single patient I interact with the same way. In order to grasp what makes every single patient or practitioner unique, I need to know everything there is to know about you. As an integrative medicine practitioner, it is essential that I gather as much data as I can in order to connect all the puzzle pieces. This is also true of the practitioners I train. Practitioners often come to me and say, "I want to learn how to do stem cell therapy," or, "I want to integrate peptides into my practice." My response is always, "Well, tell me about you, your practice, your challenges, and how you and your team interact with patients," and on and on. This information often leads to insights and clues that change the way they think of their own practices, even beyond the one or two modalities they were originally interested in.

When it comes to patients, we have a few very simple goals we try to help patients achieve, no matter the condition that they present to me in our offices:

1. Ensure optimal functionality and quality of life for the longest period of time.

2. Build a strong, genuine, altruistic relationship with the patient (or practitioners) to ensuring a lifelong partnership.

3. Ensure that our patients are educated on all facets of their health (the good and the bad) and have the information they need to make their own health decisions, based on unbiased health guidance.

4. Work toward eliminating all prescription drugs that a patient may be taking.

5. Ensure we can provide all the tools necessary for an individual to enjoy the best health outcomes and achieve their short- and long-term goals.

With every patient we work with and every practitioner we train, we attempt to take into account their short- and long-term goals. Our clinics try to build an all-inclusive ecosystem that leads to the best outcomes and maintains seamless continuity of care.

As of 2021, we are at a true crossroads in public health. The pandemic showed us in vivid terms that the current healthcare system could not keep up with demands of sick people. Now more than ever we must recognize the need for change. Let's make the COVID-19 pandemic the catalyst for the change we desperately need. Let's ensure this does not happen again and start making the shift in healthcare delivery now, so if something like this does happen again, we will be much better prepared. As much as the global pandemic has been a curse and frustrating as a practitioner, it gives me hope that people are starting to recognize the importance of what we do and how we practice medicine. It has also given much-needed awareness and raised the profile of our scope of practice.

Science, medicine, and technology continue to advance exponentially while the healthcare system continues to significantly lag, only caring about health once a problem has developed far enough along to warrant an intervention. As a healthcare practitioner, it's encouraging to see energy and passion directed toward new approaches to deliver better medical care. Moving forward, the hope is that we can build on what already works in our medical system and expand its benefits equally to everybody. The United States is already the world leader in trauma care, as well as medical technology. Our ability to treat complicated cancers is unrivaled, even though there remains a long way to go in oncology. And we are world leaders in many parts of cardiac medicine and minimally invasive procedures.

If we can take these advances and then build a more patient-centric healthcare system, we can truly deliver on the promise of good care for everyone. Patients will be at the center of this new system—at least at my clinics, they already are.

A Traditional Doctor's Change of Heart

Evelina Grayver, MD, FACC

Evelina Grayver, MD, FACC, is the definition of a traditionally trained doctor. She went to medical school before specializing in cardiology and doing her internship and residency at Northwell in New York, followed by stints as fellow and chief fellow. After her fellowship, Dr. Grayver joined the Northwell staff as director of the cardiac ICU, a remarkable honor for a young doctor fresh from her fellowship.

Working in the ICU, Dr. Grayver regularly saw the sickest cardiac patients, treating conditions like acute heart attack, end-stage heart failure, transplant patients, and patients with fatal arrhythmias. Over time, Grayver began to develop a particular interest in heart health for women, who often don't experience heart disease the same as men and are tragically under-treated in many cases. She created a women's heart health program aimed at educating women about heart disease and focusing on cardio-obstetrics.

Then COVID-19 came along and threw her working life into chaos. She was re-deployed into the COVID units, where she served through the worst summer months of 2020 as the pandemic raged. By the time she was re-deployed back to cardiology, she was wrung out.

"Living in the ICU setting took a significant toll on me, physically, mentally, and emotionally," she remembered later. "I'd been taking atrocious care of myself and allowed an inflammatory cascade to take over my body. I was drained and weak. I had zero energy and barely slept. It was the effect of all the inflammatory chemicals in my system."

Back in the cardiology unit, she was seeing young, healthy women with conditions like pre-eclampsia—and made a connection between their conditions and her own depleted state. It was all about chronic inflammation. Yet when she looked into the effects of inflammation and how to prevent it, she was shocked to realize how little traditional medicine really understood inflammation.

This is where functional medicine came in. Despite being doubted by her own colleagues, many of whom were openly dismissive of her interest in reducing inflammation to improve health, she began to read and eventually reached out to me. My approach with Dr. Grayver was the same as with all my patients: I first took the time to understand her condition with a thorough history, then ordered a comprehensive battery of tests. Even for a critical care cardiologist, the testing was comprehensive. "I'd never seen the extent of this blood work," Dr. Grayver said. "I'd never been taught to diagnose inflammatory disease."

The results of the blood work and my history came back with shocking results. Chronologically, she was forty-three years old, but her biological age was closer to fifty-eight. She was experiencing adrenal burnout, endocrine disruption that was identical to pre-menopause, and subclinical levels of multiple hormones including estrogen, progesterone, thyroid, and testosterone.

Based on these results, we designed a therapeutic program customized to her needs. It included a supplement regimen of iron, cell support, adrenal gland support, and magnesium. She also started taking bio-identical thyroid and sex hormones. The result? A dramatic and rapid improvement in Dr. Grayver's biomarkers and day-to-day quality of life.

"My colleagues say this is all mumbo jumbo," she said. "But after a month of this therapy, they were asking me, 'What are you doing? You look radiant. You have a pep in your step.'"

Her answer for this skepticism is to challenge her colleagues to look at patients who have been treated with functional medicine pre- and post-treatment. Invariably, they'll find decreased inflammatory markers, improved health, greater disease resistance, higher quality sleep, better mood, and overall improvements in quality of life.

Now an enthusiastic convert to the full scope of preventive medicine offered through functional medicine, Dr. Grayver is looking for ways to expand its reach. About 80 percent of cardiovascular disease is preventable, she says, with proper lifestyle intervention. The same applies for cancers and metabolic disease. Arresting the inflammatory cascade before advanced disease develops makes it possible for many patients to entirely avoid developing these deadly conditions.

"We need to understand the importance of preventive medicine," she said. "The good news is I think traditionally trained physicians are becoming more comfortable with the idea that a lot of diseases are caused by inflammation. They just don't know how to appropriately track it and treat it. But we're chipping away it. They're beginning to understand."

Chapter 11

Creating Smart Healthcare Consumers

"Healthcare's like any other product or service: If the consumer is in charge of spending his money on it, then the market will make sure that it is affordable."

—Rush Limbaugh

As a healthcare provider running a successful integrative medicine practice, I'm often asked three questions:

- "How and why did you get into this field?"

- "What's the best way to help patients take control of their own healthcare and earn true autonomy?"

- "I want to get out of my current conventional medicine practice. How can I set up a practice like yours?" (This last one comes from practitioners.)

Beginning with patients, it's essential to recognize first that we live in an era saturated with information. This is one of the biggest challenges we face, but also one of the greatest positives. Today, consumers have unlimited access to a huge amount of health information. Some of it, from sites like WebMD and the Mayo Clinic site, is solid and accurate, but often doesn't include the full range of what we know and too often steers people in a certain direction.

These sites are the bastion of traditional medicine and tend to ignore many of the therapies we successfully use to treat thousands of patients. Additionally, they rely on generalized reference ranges that are often too conservative or recommend "normal" reference ranges that are unacceptable. Finally, they tend to promote conventional options, such as drugs and surgery, for conditions we know can be treated with education and lifestyle modification.

Take cholesterol as a high-profile example. On virtually every page dealing with cholesterol on their site, WebMD prominently recommends statin medications, often in the same sentence as diet and exercise. The overall impression is that statin medications are at the same risk and effectiveness level as diet and exercise. There are a number of problems with this approach. There may be a place for statin medications in the context of high cholesterol, but they should not be a first-line treatment. As effective as they may be for some people, statin medications are pharmaceuticals and have well-documented side effects ranging from minor to very serious. Also, a statin medication is a highly targeted therapy that's designed to do only one primary thing: reduce LDL cholesterol levels. In most people, however, issues aren't just limited to elevated LDL cholesterol. If a patient's LDL cholesterol is elevated because of other factors like insulin resistance, hormone imbalance, or metabolic syndrome, what good will a statin do? It can't address any of these underlying conditions.

As a healthcare provider concerned about the whole patient, it's important that I view elevated LDL in the context of that patient's overall health. What is their diet like? Are they overweight? Do they have symptoms of other conditions that may be signaling some underlying disease process? What is their inflammatory burden? Do they consume a lot of healthy fats like avocados, fish, and nuts? Once I know the answers to these questions, along with their LDL number, I can design a comprehensive, whole-health treatment plan that will most likely correct the LDL numbers on the way to better overall health and quality of life. This approach makes much more sense to me than just writing an prescription for a statin that will most likely cause muscle and joint aches, lower good HDL cholesterol, and deplete the body of one of the most essential substances in the body, coenzyme-Q 10!

However, even with the drawbacks associated with these big sites, patients who have researched their health on sites like WebMD and Mayo Clinic often walk into our clinic with a better grounding in basic medical terms and concepts, and that's a positive thing. It gives us a chance to build on their knowledge base and expand it.

The next issue, unfortunately, is that too often patients don't know how to distinguish between the solid but somewhat flawed information they can find on a site like the Mayo Clinic and the tsunami of bad information that is presented next to it. Some of this is due to the way the Internet search engines work, especially Google. When a patient types "high cholesterol treatment" into Google, the results are a mixed bag of good sites, paid advertisements, and high-ranking garbage articles from sites that have figured out how to game Google's search results but aren't concerned about presenting high-quality information. The advertisements, in particular, are suspect: these come from companies that can afford to "buy" search ranking, no matter how effective their treatment is. The ads are almost indistinguishable from higher-quality websites and sit above those better sites on the page. In fact, you may have to scroll down once or twice to get to high-quality search results, first moving past sites pushing a whole host of dubious approaches. If a patient isn't grounded in health information, how would they know to distinguish between a site pushing a quack remedy, a site that puts medications on the same level as lifestyle modification, and a truly high-quality site that offers sound information?

It's also important to recognize that search engines and social medica platforms often restrict information on many of the therapies that we stand behind because they are not FDA approved or they are considered investigational. I regularly have meetings with our administrative team, and they tell me story after story about how social media platforms and search engines will not allow us to publish information on certain integrative medicine treatment therapies, such has hormone optimizing or stem cell therapy. Last time I checked, we have a First Amendment right to freedom of speech. All I'm trying to do is educate people on medicine and science, but these non-medical search engines and social media platforms effectively censor our ability to get good health information on so-called alternative therapies out to people.

At the end of the day, healthcare consumers need to understand that the Internet is not really their friend. Google and other search engines are primarily concerned with making money. Credibility runs second to profit. By the time a patient gets into their healthcare provider's office, they may have read pages of information that only confused them about what high cholesterol is and how it can be treated. If the practitioner is working for a traditional clinic, it's likely they won't have much time to go through all of this information in a detailed way. Instead, the patient is likely to get a few minutes of hazy talk about "losing weight" or "eating healthy" and go home with a prescription for statin medications. If they happen to have read one of the big, credible sites like Mayo, this will make perfect sense. After all, medications are the same as diet as exercise, remember?

Helping Practitioners Help Patients

This brings me to the third question I posed at the beginning of this chapter: how to form a practice that creates educated patients and offers comprehensive preventative care. Before diving in, I wanted to reinforce a few points about the all-important philosophy behind my practice. My approach to medicine is based on providing the patient with all of the knowledge and tools they need to make healthy decisions for themselves, point blank. Rather than advocating for particular treatments based on how profitable they are or my own feelings for them, I believe in presenting both sides of every question. When talking to patients about their options, my job is to relay data and the results of clinical experience, to explain both the potential upside and the potential risks of any particular treatment. A good practitioner will always present the information, the good and the bad, and let patients make their own decisions. If patients decide to do something I don't agree with 100 percent, I believe it's my job to support the patient in their approach and give them options for how to minimize any side effects or issues. A good example of this is birth control pills. I don't discourage women from being on birth control, as I understand the necessity for this therapy in certain circumstances, but I do help them to think about the long-term effects and how to minimize them, or how to support their bodies while utilizing birth control.

This is one of the areas that I spend a lot of time dealing with. Although there is an absolute time and place where things like birth control therapies are needed, patients need to understand their long-term risks, such as blood clots, heart attack, stroke, and cancer, all of which have been validated by some of the largest, best-designed clinical studies in medical history.* Again, I am not a contrarian, anti-pharma dictator, but women

---

* https://jamanetwork.com/journals/jama/fullarticle/195120.

need to understand the potential long-term risks when using these types of therapies. If a woman decides she would like to use an oral contraceptive, we pivot our conversation toward what we can do to help minimize any long-term or short-term side effects and help her body work as well as it can. Although many women don't know it, there are adjunctive therapies we use every day to help minimize the long-term negative risks of oral contraceptives without decreasing efficacies of the oral contraceptive.

My approach to care is grounded in the idea that medicine needs to be intensely personal and individualized. Every patient is unique, with unique needs and a unique history and life circumstances. Every patient has different short- and long-term goals. It's impossible to really learn about patients in a five-minute visit every six months. At our clinics, regardless of a patient's age, pre-existing conditions, or lifestyle, we see all patients at an absolute bare minimum of twice per year, and that would be for a healthy thirty-year-old with a clean lifestyle and no major health issues. A majority of our patients, however, come in on a quarterly basis for a full in-depth consultation and comprehensive work-up, including the all-important blood work. We look at the metrics that are essential to the prophylactic practice of medicine, such as inflammatory markers, hormones, adrenal markers, heavy metals, autoimmune markers, macro- and micronutrients, neurotransmitters, gut parameters, cancer markers, and telomere length. These are some of the things we need to monitor to identify changes early so we can be more proactive than reactive. This is how we should all be practicing and consuming medicine.

Not surprisingly, this intensive level of care is one of the biggest changes most healthcare providers face when they transition to a functional and integrative approach. Instead of seeing forty patients a day, providers can expect to see ten patients but spend more time with each of them, plus extra time following up. The advantages to this approach are obvious: a better understanding of each patient and improved continuity of care. The communication is more consistent between visits and from year to year. The result is patients who not only benefit from better care, but who feel heard and have a much better understanding of their own health and choices.

The next issue that frequently comes up is the scope of practice. Practices like mine are frequently cash-based, fee-for-service practices that accept little or no reimbursement from insurance companies. This is an important point for several reasons but most importantly is a huge barrier to entry for many patients to seeing us. Many patients fear that an integrative medicine clinic will cost "too much" for them to maintain so they don't even bother coming in. Or hesitate as "these types of clinics are only for the rich and elite" and never bother to call. In today's fee-for-service clinic world, a lot of practitioners have decided an easy way to make money is to specialize in one or two procedures. This makes sense from a purely business perspective—it's easier to advertise an infusion clinic or hormone-replacement clinic online than it is to advertise a more comprehensive but less well-defined practice. The issue, however, is that these single-focus clinics can't possibly consider a patient's full health needs. To a hormone replacement clinic, everything is going to look like a hormone deficiency. To an infusion clinic, there's nothing that can't be fixed with an infusion. Patients end up getting short-changed and under-treated.

Unfortunately, I see this all the time from patients who come to our clinics after wasting so much time and money and not getting any results from more narrow-focused alternative medicine practices. These bad experiences bias the patient against alternative approaches, which makes the problem worse. Now they don't want to try another integrative medicine practice, fully believing there is no way they can be helped, so they ultimately just go back to what their conventional practitioner says. Then, back in their "regular" doctor's office, they repeat their bad experience, which only reinforces the conventional practitioner's outlook that alternative therapies are a waste of time and money. And the cycle goes on ever repeating.

On the opposite end of the spectrum, sometimes fee-for-service clinics have unrealistic perspectives on the average American's financial wherewithal and price services beyond the reach of most people. I am sure you have heard of concierge medicine programs and think this is a concept that only the rich and famous can benefit from. This may be the case for some high-end concierge medical practices, but in reality all medicine should be "concierge." Healthcare practitioners have an innate responsibility to service our patients to the best of our ability, regardless of compensation. Practices like ours ensure that we deliver the highest quality of care without requiring that patients make six figures to afford it. Everyone needs concierge-style individualized care without needing to be a millionaire! The concept of personalized healthcare with attention to detail, empathy, and compassion is the way medicine should always be practiced.

The other challenge facing fee-for-service practices comes from patients themselves. More than 90 percent of people in the United States have some form of health insurance, including tens of millions of people paying for expensive private plans.* When confronted with a fee-for-service practice that's not covered under their existing plan, these patients will

---

* Census Bureau. Health insurance: coverage in the United States: 2019. census.gov/library/publications/2020/demo/p60-271.html.

understandably balk since they are already paying for basic care (or at least assume they are).

At the same time, there is a widespread perception that fee-for-service medical care is too expensive. This idea is reinforced by news stories of outrageous medical bills. The overwhelming perception in the United States is that medical care is extremely expensive. And the situation is made worse by unscrupulous fee-for-service practices that charge very high consultation fees. Unfortunately, I know firsthand of prominent health care providers in my scope of practice who charge $500 or even more for a single consultation. Not only is this unnecessarily expensive, it casts the entire functional medicine world in a bad light by making it seem as if we are all profiteering.

While these are significant challenges to any functional medicine practice, they can be overcome with a strategic plan and good communication. At my clinic, we hold the cost of the initial visit down, and we quickly prove the value of our care through results and intensely personal care. There is a qualitative difference in the level of care a patient receives at a well-run functional medicine clinic and a busy traditional practice governed by insurance regulations. Our patients get more face-to-face time with qualified healthcare providers and receive highly personalized care, coupled with intensive education. Also, good clinics should have programs in place to make sure that money is never an obstacle to good care. This may involve payment programs, loans, or other tools to ensure that patients from every walk of life can get premium medical care.

Even with all these measures in place, however, there will always be the question of private insurance to deal with. The fact is that insurance won't cover many of the therapies we recommend, and I'm not sure I would welcome insurance companies into my practice even if they did because insurance is a double-edged sword. If they started approving our type of practices, it would drive in more business, but it would enable insurance companies and governing agencies to tell us what we can and can't do. Once a practice starts billing insurance, it introduces a third party into the provider/patient relationship. I like the thought of accepting insurance, but I don't know if it can be executed in the best interest of the patient, which ultimately is the only thing that matters.

Rethink Private Health Insurance

So, what's the best option? As radical as it may sound, I don't advocate for private health insurance for many patients—and I live by these words in my own life. My own family is only covered by a catastrophic insurance policy that will protect us in the event of a major illness or accident. For ongoing, routine medical care, we pay cash out of pocket. This approach makes sense to me, because major illnesses and accidents can be devastatingly expensive, but they are also relatively rare. This means catastrophic insurance policies are much less expensive, because you're much less likely to actually use the insurance. However, if you do need it, it's there, so patients don't have to worry about going bankrupt because of a car accident or sudden, serious illness like COVID-19.

Once we remove private, comprehensive insurance from the equation, it begins to make more sense. Here's a real-world example of how this works. I recently got insurance quotes for myself, a healthy thirty-three-year-old man with a super clean diet and lifestyle. I was quoted a policy with $5,000 annual deductible and $500/month payments. This just isn't reasonable for the level of care I need, so I ended up ditching the idea of comprehensive health insurance and buying an acute-care policy.

This option was clear to me, but in my experience, the average middle-class family is so spooked by the high cost of medical care that going without insurance is unthinkable. It takes a significant amount of time to explain that dropping expensive monthly insurance that won't cover the basics in favor of a catastrophic policy and fee-for-service treatments actually saves money—but this is time well-spent. In the end, my patients who choose to go this route end up with better medical care at less cost, considering that our fee for an office visit is about $150, or around a quarter of what most families would expect to pay for a single month's coverage under traditional insurance.

As we're discussing changing the healthcare paradigm, this is a good time to look at the ways it's already changing and how that will affect the patient/provider relationship. Over 2020, as the coronavirus pandemic has

---

Many patients feel uncomfortable with just having acute care insurance. But they need to see the numbers. They might already be spending $5,000 a year on co-pays and drugs, but if they see that all they need is acute coverage and spend the rest of that money on functional, preventive care, they'll have a better quality of life and a longer life.

—Evelina Grayver, MD, FACC
Director of Women's Heart Health, Northwell Central Region and
Katz Women's Institute

swept the world, the entire healthcare industry was forced into a period of rapid change. This was shocking to many, because healthcare is traditionally a very slow business to change—it can take decades for evidence-based changes in practice to be widely adopted, and don't even get started on the widespread use of antiquated technologies like fax machines to transmit patient information.

The change, however, was essential, because the virus not only promised to strain our healthcare system to the breaking point, it also created a situation where tens of millions of people were afraid to go into their doctor's offices for routine visits. According to the CDC, by the fall of 2020, as many as 41 percent of Americans had delayed some kind of medical care, including 12 percent that delayed urgent care of serious conditions.* As a result of this fear, telemedicine boomed as healthcare providers and their patients turned to a safe, distanced form of communication.

Despite the grim reasons for this change, it was interesting to me as a healthcare provider, as we've been using telemedicine for years to reach patients. In fact, one of the ways we are able to hold costs down is by prescribing treatments that can be self-administered and teaching patients how to administer it themselves at home. This is true for micronutrient and hormone balancing therapies. We've been using telemedicine for years with this type of therapy, which makes it possible for us to follow our patients all over the world and provide them access to top-notch information and care.

This proves that the way we have been delivering healthcare to our patients for over ten years has always been the best delivery system, and I'm glad conventional healthcare is finally starting to back the adoption of telemedicine. I'm finally starting to see widespread discussion of things like vitamin C, zinc, and vitamin D3 to help prevent serious illness.

In the future, I expect to see this trend toward remote medicine accelerating. I also expect that functional medicine will continue to make inroads—there's already a huge demand for our type of care model, and it's still growing. As more patients experience the difference between a traditional turn-and-burn approach and the kind of intensely personalized care they can receive at a well-run clinic, we expect to see more and more people breaking out of the traditional mold and taking control of their healthcare, even when it means abandoning their traditional insurance plans. Our goal as healthcare providers is to help patients make this transition as seamless as possible, so once again, it goes back to our role as health

---

* Centers for Disease Control and Prevention. Delay or avoidance of medical care because of COVID-19–related concerns. https://www.cdc.gov/mmwr/volumes/69/wr/mm6936a4.htm.

educators. In this case, however, it's about more than providing accurate information about treatments and therapies. Instead, we are increasingly tasked with providing patients a roadmap to better care at less cost and giving them the knowledge and tools to make healthy choices that will radically improve their quality of life, extend lifespan, and reduce their risk of getting serious disease.

This is the future we are working toward, and despite the many serious challenges we face in medicine, I'm very confident this is the future that will happen—but we'll need patients to hold us accountable. As healthcare providers, we all swore a Hippocratic oath to "first do no harm" when we started practicing. The oath boils down to avoiding the knife and letting the body heal itself. Unfortunately, we as healthcare practitioners often know that the way most of the world practices medicine is wrong. We know we are in violation of our sacred Hippocratic oath. We must be held responsible. We need to go back to understanding what Hippocrates wrote about in his famous oath:

> I swear to fulfill, to the best of my ability and judgment, this covenant:
>
> I will respect the hard-won scientific gains of those physicians in whose steps I walk, and gladly share such knowledge as is mine with those who are to follow.
>
> I will apply, for the benefit of the sick, all measures [that] are required, avoiding those twin traps of overtreatment and therapeutic nihilism.
>
> I will remember that there is art to medicine as well as science, and that warmth, sympathy, and understanding may outweigh the surgeon's knife or the chemist's drug.
>
> I will not be ashamed to say "I know not," nor will I fail to call in my colleagues when the skills of another are needed for a patient's recovery.
>
> I will respect the privacy of my patients, for their problems are not disclosed to me that the world may know. Most especially must I tread with care in matters of life and death. If it is given me to save a life, all thanks. But it may also be within my power to take a life; this awesome responsibility must be faced with great humbleness

and awareness of my own frailty. Above all, I must not play at God.

I will remember that I do not treat a fever chart, a cancerous growth, but a sick human being, whose illness may affect the person's family and economic stability. My responsibility includes these related problems, if I am to care adequately for the sick.

I will prevent disease whenever I can, for prevention is preferable to cure.

I will remember that I remain a member of society, with special obligations to all my fellow human beings, those sound of mind and body as well as the infirm.

If I do not violate this oath, may I enjoy life and art, respected while I live and remembered with affection thereafter. May I always act so as to preserve the finest traditions of my calling, and may I long experience the joy of healing those who seek my help.

After reading that, can you say that your healthcare provider follows all those guidelines?

Does your practitioner deliver on this promise? Does healthcare in this country live and operate by these standards?

PART THREE
TAKE CONTROL OF AGING

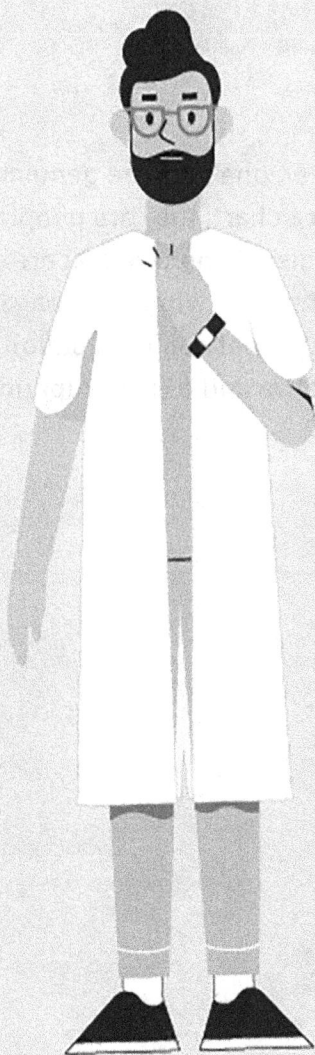

GENUINE

To be a good healer, one must be genuine. Patients are not just a name on a chart; they are people able to detect inauthenticity. By displaying true sincere care, providers are more likely to break the white coat barrier with patients and have open and honest communication that will lead to more effective and overall superior care.

Chapter 12

Understanding Aging

"*The medicine for anti-aging is lifelong learning.*"

—**Robin Sharma**

For the final chapters, I want to dive into one of the most exciting areas of medicine today: anti-aging and regenerative medicine, including the good, the bad, the misconceptions, and why you need to think about anti-aging medicine, even when you're young!

Not too long ago (and somewhat still to this day), the very concept of "anti-aging medicine" was mocked within traditional healthcare and the media. The idea of aging, gradually growing more frail and sicker until we finally succumb, was considered as immutable as the speed of light or the presence of gravity. The concept of aging and the fear of death has been baked into every culture's self-awareness since the first humans picked up a chisel to carve hieroglyphics into stone. Immortality was reserved for gods and science fiction.

Beginning around the 1980s, however, a number of pioneering scientists began to look at aging not as a law of nature but as a series of processes that could be understood. We began to understand the underlying cellular and molecular mechanisms that drive aging, everything from the rate of cell division and cell death to the health of the microbiome in the gut and how it affects tissue health. Slowly, a consensus began to emerge that not only was aging a process that could be understood, it was a process that in some cases could be dramatically slowed or even reversed.

Nowhere is this more obvious than in so-called "blue zones." First popularized by a team of writers from *National Geographic* magazine, blue zones are areas in the world where people enjoy an unusually long and health lifespan. Blue zones have been identified in far-flung communities, including Loma Linda, California; Nicoya, Costa Rica, Sardinia, Italy; Ikaria, Greece; and Okinawa, Japan. In each of these areas—despite dramatically different cultural backgrounds and even climates—people reached the age of one hundred at ten times greater rates than in the United States. Moreover, they were healthier, suffering from less diabetes, heart disease, liver and lung disease, and even cancer. So, what was it about these particular areas that led people to live longer?

It turned out the answer was deceptively simple: the people in these blue zones led healthier lives. They walked a lot throughout the day. They led less stressful lives. They ate mostly plant-based diets rich in whole grains and fresh, seasonal vegetables, complemented by foods high in healthy fats like fatty fish. And they enjoyed a strong sense of community and social support.*

While only a small percentage of people actually live in blue zones, scientists began to pursue research hoping to apply the lessons they had learned about living a longer, healthier life to everyday life. Some of the earliest successes in evidence-based anti-aging medicine came from calorie restriction, or the practice of severely limiting calories to prolong lifespan. The theory behind calorie restriction was basic: if you imagine the body as a car, then eating and digesting are similar to driving and gassing up your care—in other words, it's wear and tear. The theory is that, by eating and digesting less, the body is subjected to less wear and tear and fewer insults from unhealthy food.

Early research bore this theory out in every animal model it was tested. Calorie restriction was shown to result in dramatically improved glucose levels, blood pressure, cholesterol levels, and other markers of aging. In short-lived animals like worms and rats, calorie restriction was shown to extend lifespan, in some cases by 40 percent. Spurred by these results, groups launched studies of longer-lived rhesus monkeys to see if cutting their overall calories by 30 percent would affect their longevity. After twenty years, one group of researchers reported that the monkeys did

---

* Buettner D, Skemp S. Blue zones: lessons from the world's longest lived. *Am J Lifestyle Med.* 2016;10(5):318-321. Published 2016 Jul 7. doi:10.1177/1559827616637066.

experience a longer lifespan, while the other found that the monkeys were healthier but didn't live any longer. Researchers, however, cautioned about reading too much into these results, as many of the monkeys in the studies were still alive so it was hard to draw broad conclusions.*

In humans, we're still waiting to see if calorie restriction can extend lifespan. A hardy group of people involved in the CR Forum, a global group of calorie restriction enthusiasts, has been following the program for years and regularly report excellent blood pressure, glucose control, cholesterol, and other markers of aging. However, because calorie restriction is still fairly new, and humans live so long, it will realistically be several decades before we learn how much benefit there is to people. The oldest person known to history was a Frenchwoman named Jeanne Louise Calment, who lived to the astonishing age of 122.† Who knows if someday in the future we'll meet calorie restriction pioneers living far beyond 122 years, to reach some theoretical maximum of human age?

In the meantime, the practice of intermittent fasting has gained widespread adoption. In this practice, instead of fully limiting calories around the clock, people alternate periods of fasting or calorie reduction with more traditional eating patterns. Think of it like "calorie-restriction light." According to Harvard Medical School, there's a "ton of promising intermittent fasting" research. If the fasting periods are timed correctly with the circadian cycle, the practice helps people lose weight but also dramatically improves markers of aging like blood glucose.‡ In part, intermittent fasting works because it stresses the cells. We're used to thinking of stress in a negative sense, but in this case, the stress of fasting has powerful benefits for cells, similar to exercise. Vigorous exercise stresses muscles and the cardiovascular system, prompting them to rebuild better. Intermittent fasting does something similar, stressing cells and prompting them to function more efficiently. As long as you support your body, live in a nurturing environment, and give your body time to recover, it will grow stronger.§

As promising as calorie restriction and intermittent fasting are, it turns out this was only the beginning of a torrent of research that sought to unravel the mysteries of aging. At first ridiculed, there's no longer any

---

* U.S. Department of Health and Human Services. Calorie restriction and fasting diets: what do we know? https://www.nia.nih.gov/health/calorie-restriction-and-fasting-diets-what-do-we-know#animal.
† Wikipedia. Jeanne Calment. https://en.wikipedia.org/wiki/Jeanne_Calment.
‡ Harvard Health Publishing, Harvard Medical School. Intermittent fasting: surprising update. https://www.health.harvard.edu/blog/intermittent-fasting-surprising-update-2018062914156.
§ Collier R. Intermittent fasting: the science of going without. *CMAJ.* 2013;185(9):E363-E364. doi: 10.1503/cmaj.109-4451.

doubt that we are making major breakthroughs in anti-aging medicine. A new branch of medicine I discussed in the last chapter, regenerative medicine, draws heavily on anti-aging research and seeks to reverse or slow aging in tissues and cells. Similarly, many of the concepts in this book also slow aging, including following certain lifestyle practices that have been well-documented to slow or inhibit cellular aging. Remember, our bodies are kinetic "chains," and any chain is only as good as its weakest link! But if we address every link in the health chain, our bodies can function optimally—ensuring the slowing or reversing of the aging process!

Before we dive into anti-aging medicine, however, it's important to first understand what aging is and how it works. As strange as this may seem, both medicine and our general culture profoundly misunderstand aging. Conventional medical practitioners tend to treat aging and the diseases that come along with it as inevitabilities that may be temporarily slowed with medications, while our culture treats aging as if it's only skin-deep and can be treated with a little bit of Botox and some moisturizing lotion.

Unfortunately, neither of these positions really helps anybody. By treating aging and the diseases of aging like a foregone conclusion, too many people are conditioned into accepting the decline in their health as something they're helpless to fix. Instead of actively working to prevent or even reverse the underlying conditions that are causing these diseases, they are trained to wait until it's harder to make major improvements in their lives. And by focusing exclusively on the outward aspects of aging—the wrinkled skin and thinning hair—our culture confuses people about what aging is and leads people to believe that aging is only represented by wrinkles and droopy skin.

So, what should we be paying attention to? As I've said before, it's all about what's going on inside your body.

What Is Aging?

Let's step back and look at the very basic question: What is aging? Once we understand what aging actually is, and what it isn't, it becomes much easier to identify therapies and interventions that target aging itself.

I'll begin with a negative—what aging is not. Aging is not a disease. It is not cancer, heart disease, or diabetes. Although these are all more common among older people, these dreaded diseases are better understood as "diseases of aging." They are caused in many cases by the underlying processes of aging and are only the most outward and last steps in destructive processes that usually are in place for decades before the problem becomes obvious. This distinction between aging itself and the diseases of aging is critical to understand, because it allows us to build a philosophical framework to understand and confront the aging processes themselves.

Aging is best understood as a time-dependent process during which the basic function of your cells and body undergo gradual changes. These changes are uneven—time doesn't affect all of your organ systems at the same rate, or in the same way. It's entirely possible to suffer from atherosclerotic arteries thanks to years of plaque build-up while enjoying a robust immune system. In this way, we have to think of aging as two distinct phenomena: there is chronological age, which is measured by the number of birthdays you tick off a calendar, and there is biological age, which is a measure of how much wear and tear your organs have experienced. If you've ever met someone in their seventies who seems to glow with vibrant health, you've already seen with your eyes that biological age and chronological age can be radically different.

Here's the good news: unless you have a time machine, you can't affect chronological age. Time is time. But chronological age isn't the one most people should care about. Instead, biological age is the critical measure we should be tracking. What really matters is how our organs are functioning—a fifty-year-old who has a massive heart attack thanks to advanced coronary disease doesn't much care what her chronological age is. What matters most is the biological age of her arteries. The same is true for the thirty-year-old woman with the imbalanced hormone levels of a postmenopausal sixty-year-old woman. Imagine how a thirty-year-old body is performing when she has hormone levels of a sixty-year-old biologically.

Once we start looking at biological age, especially with the understanding that organ systems age at different rates, the entire concept of age and aging begins to shift into focus. We start to see aging not as the relentless countdown of minutes and hours until death. Instead, we can view aging as a group of separate processes happening in organs throughout the body, each operating at a different speed and influenced by different factors. This is the framework that anti-aging researchers and practitioners are using, and they've already made great progress in understanding how different organ systems are affected by factors of aging: inflammation, DNA breakdown and cell senescence, the environment, stress, and lifestyle choices like diet and exercise.

Inflammation

I touched on this in an earlier chapter, but it's worth revisiting inflammation in the context of aging. Chronic inflammation may be the single most damaging factor when it comes to long-term disease and the most influential factor when it comes to the aging process. Remember that chronic inflammation is not the type that makes your joints swell after injury (although it does do that as well!). We're talking about cellular inflammation, or the process of inhibiting cellular mitochondria function and activity. Inflammation has the ability to affect any organ system, including our physical and cognitive systems. All of our most dreaded diseases, including heart disease, have inflammation at its roots—and we are still learning more about the many ways inflammation affects our biology. Just a few examples include:

- Chronic inflammation was directly linked to increased risk of heart attack and stroke, according to research published by Johns Hopkins. This effect was true whether or not cholesterol levels were elevated—inflammation itself was the culprit.*

- We are experiencing a rapid increase in the number of people suffering from autoimmune diseases, thanks in part to chronic inflammation. This includes rheumatoid arthritis, ulcerative colitis and Crohn's disease, complications of type 2 diabetes (we are increasingly learning that type 2 diabetes has an autoimmune component), asthma, dermatological conditions, and many others. In each of these cases, the presence of inflammatory factors at the disease site aggravates the condition and contributes to symptoms.

- Chronic inflammation in the gut is linked directly to diseases like inflammatory bowel disease and ulcers. Gut health is intimately related to the level of inflammation.

- New research is breaking ground on the role of chronic inflammation in depression and other mental health conditions. It turns out that low-level inflammation activates the immune system in a way that contributes to the production and function

---

* Johns Hopkins Medicine. Fight inflammation to help prevent heart disease. https://www.hopkins-medicine.org/health/wellness-and-prevention/fight-inflammation-to-help-prevent-heart-disease.

of neurotransmitters and, through increased oxidative stress, makes depression worse.*

- Neurological conditions like Parkinson's disease and even Alzheimer's, where inflammatory chemicals have been shown to attack the damaged brain cells that are already weakened or aged. Researchers currently believe that inflammation may make symptoms associated with these diseases dramatically worse.†

There are many more such examples, but the point is clear: chronic inflammation is incredibly dangerous and poses a serious threat throughout the body.

What Causes Inflammation?

We've discussed the difference between acute inflammation and chronic inflammation, but it's worth a quick review. Acute inflammation is the localized immune system response that occurs in response to a direct injury, like the swelling that happens after you burn your finger or cut yourself. Chronic inflammation, however, occurs when the immune system is activated at a low level, flooding the body with dangerous inflammatory chemicals, cytokines, and chemokines that damage cells and tissues.

Why would this happen? What are the driving factors that underlie so much chronic inflammation?

In most cases, the answer is depressingly obvious and preventable. The leading causes of chronic inflammation are poor diet, stress, lack of sleep, and exposure to environmental toxins. The unfortunate truth is that we live in a pro-inflammatory culture—it's virtually impossible to eliminate exposure to inflammatory factors in day-to-day life. And we can't just blame our genetics or our busy schedules! We know that lifestyle decisions can overcome genetic predispositions. It turns out that DNA is *not* destiny.

---

* Berk, M, Williams, LJ, Jacka, FN et al. So depression is an inflammatory disease, but where does the inflammation come from?. *BMC Med* 11, 200 (2013). https://doi.org/10.1186/1741-7015-11-200.
† Akiyama H, Barger S, Barnum S, Bradt B, Bauer J, Cole GM, Cooper NR, Eikelenboom P, Emmerling M, Fiebich BL, Finch CE, Frautschy S, Griffin WS, Hampel H, Hull M, Landreth G, Lue L, Mrak R, Mackenzie IR, McGeer PL, O'Banion MK, Pachter J, Pasinetti G, Plata-Salaman C, Rogers J, Rydel R, Shen Y, Streit W, Strohmeyer R, Tooyoma I, Van Muiswinkel FL, Veerhuis R, Walker D, Webster S, Wegrzyniak B, Wenk G, Wyss-Coray T. Inflammation and Alzheimer's disease. *Neurobiol Aging.* 2000 May-Jun;21(3):383-421. doi: 10.1016/s0197-4580(00)00124-x. PMID: 10858586; PMCID: PMC3887148.

All these diets confuse the issue. People think they should eat more on a keto diet, so they eat bacon and salami. You see people on all these wacky diets, but each fad diet takes us further away from a healthy diet.

—**Elyse Marrone, Clinical Director**
Lifestyle Nutrition Institute

The pro-inflammatory problems begin in the grocery store, where our foods are loaded with pro-inflammatory ingredients that preserve shelf-life but are highly dangerous for humans to consume. Our modern food supply, with its focus on sugar, salt, and fat may as well have been designed in a lab to kill people. It encourages obesity, which is linked to a multitude of diseases, and doesn't make any room for healthy food choices. The proper term to describe our food environment is "obesogenic," meaning that we are literally surrounded by obesity-causing messages and foods all day, every day.

One of the worst dietary culprits is unhealthy fat. Until very recently, you could walk into any grocery store and find dozens of products loaded with trans fat, a formerly common ingredient in all sorts of baked goods. This type of fat has absolutely no nutritive value and doesn't exist in nature anywhere. It's a lab-made solid fat that goes straight to the arteries. As a result, it was banned from the U.S. food supply in 2018—after decades of polluting arteries.* In place of trans fats, however, the food industry took only a half-step toward health and now relies on saturated fats to keep food lasting longer and tasting better. Saturated fats are unhealthy fats that contribute to disease and should be consumed in moderation. They are commonly found in full-fat dairy products, red meat, and processed snacks.

Unhealthy fats aren't the only culprit. Sugar in all of its forms is highly inflammatory—and our entire food supply is drenched in sugar. In recent years, there's been a movement away from corn syrup thanks to a growing awareness of how dangerous this simple sugar is. But what was it replaced with? Cane sugar, beet sugar, raw sugar...in other words, all we've done is swap one type of sugar for another. This has occurred even as health authorities sound ever-increasing alarms on the amount of sugar people are eating and how it affects health. According to research published by

---

* Harvard Health Publishing. The truth about fats: the good, the bad, and the in-between. https://www.health.harvard.edu/staying-healthy/the-truth-about-fats-bad-and-good.

Harvard University, sugar is linked to metabolic disorders liked diabetes, cardiovascular disease, cancer, obesity, and more.*

Along with unhealthy fats and sugar, the third leg of the unhealthy food stool is salt, which is directly linked to high blood pressure and inflammation. Processed foods, pre-prepared foods, and restaurants foods are loaded with a shocking amount of salt. According to the American Heart Association, the average adult should aim to eat about 1,500 mg of salt per day.† To put that into perspective, that's about one teaspoon of salt per day, total. When you consider that a single can of soup has about 700 mg of salt and a 3-ounce serving of deli ham has about 1,100, it becomes clear how much extra salt most adults are eating, with dire health consequences.‡

Beyond excessive fat, salt, sugar, the rest of our food supply is loaded with even more pro-inflammatory foods, including gluten, dairy, alcohol, caffeine, and processed and overcooked meats. And the problems go even further up the food chain to the way food itself is produced, even "healthy foods." Our current agribusiness model relies on producing the most food at the lowest cost possible. This translates into animals that are pumped full of antibiotics to increase meat and milk production, vegetables and fruits that are genetically modified and spend their lives drenched in herbicides and pesticides, and a food supply that is laden with hormones and estrogenic compounds. All of this, of course, is approved by the government agencies that are supposed to be protecting us. How can a regular person make good decisions when there are billions of dollars of regulatory and marketing interests aligned against them?

Diet, of course, isn't the only pro-inflammatory pressure weighing on us. Stress and lack of sleep—which are both common in a normal year and skyrocketed during the COVID-19 pandemic that swept the United States—also contribute to inflammation and encourage disease. In fact, there are many, many causes of inflammation beyond diet, stress, and lack of sleep. It's fair to say most of us live in pro-inflammatory environment.

Controlling Inflammation

The depth of the problem with inflammation can be discouraging. If we live in a culture that is soaked in inflammatory factors, and encourages us

---

* Harvard Health Publishing. The sweet danger of sugar. https://www.health.harvard.edu/heart-health/the-sweet-danger-of-sugar.
† American Heart Association. How much sodium should I eat per day? https://www.heart.org/en/healthy-living/healthy-eating/eat-smart/sodium/how-much-sodium-should-i-eat-per-day.
‡ Healthline. 30 foods high in sodium. https://www.healthline.com/nutrition/foods-high-in-sodium.

at every turn to continue living dangerously, what hope is there to get it under control?

The good news is that we have more knowledge and tools than ever before. First, we are better able to measure chronic inflammation than we have been in the past. Simple blood tests for pro-inflammatory markers like C-reactive protein (CRP), plasma viscosity (PV), homocysteine, lipoprotein-A or Lp(a), and the erythrocyte sedimentation rate (ESR) can help shed light on a patient's overall inflammatory burden. The only caveat is that measuring these once or twice a year is not enough to really understand what's going on. For a truly effective anti-inflammation program to work, these should be tracked quarterly so you can adjust the care plan based on how the progress and individual are changing.

Once tracking is in place, there are a multitude of steps patients can take to control chronic inflammation, and it begins with lifestyle. In today's medical "industry," it's a problem that healthcare providers don't often have enough time to really educate patients about lifestyle interventions, because that's exactly where most health and wellness programs need to start. By adopting an anti-inflammatory lifestyle, patients can dramatically reduce their risk of disease and live longer. This means:

- Eating a healthy diet full of whole grains, bright and colorful vegetables, and healthy fats like those found in cold-water fish.

- Using supplements under the guidance of a qualified healthcare provider to address deficiencies or protect against disease.

- Limiting or eliminating alcohol and dairy consumption.

- Getting enough quality sleep every night to replenish and heal.

- Reducing extra stressors wherever possible.

- Getting enough exercise to prevent weight gain, maintain cardiovascular health, and stay strong and flexible.

But there's a catch. Sometimes even if the stars align and you have a very proactive provider and eat healthy and make good health decisions, it still may not be enough. Just because you think you're doing something healthy, it does not mean it's right for you! And just because you "feel fine" does not mean things are fine—there can be cellular changes happening that may not be significant enough to be felt. We see this frequently in our clinics. Patients come in talking about their "healthy diets" focused on foods like avocadoes, kale, and beets, but they still struggle with elevated lipids and insulin, GI concerns, inflammation, and metabolism issues. Well, guess what? Sometimes even being "healthy" may not be right for you or your body! It takes a truly comprehensive assessment to help patients identify things that are theoretically healthy but not right for their unique body. We regularly help patients identify foods and other environmental factors that just don't work for them, even if they may be healthy for other people. It's vital that, working with truly involved healthcare providers, patients learn to understand their own unique physiology and body and fight inflammation in the way that works for them.

Assaulting DNA

It's impossible to consider aging and anti-aging without looking at DNA health. In a healthy cell, DNA codes what that cell's purpose is and dictates when it will divide and eventually die. As mentioned before, this internal clock is managed by telomeres, which act as a kind of countdown clock measuring the cell's lifespan.

A healthy cell lifecycle is critical to overall health. In a normal, healthy cell, the cell is created from division or specialization into a particular type of cell (e.g., muscle, bone, blood) and performs whatever duty it was designed for. Over time, as the cell ages, it reaches a point when it divides into new cells. With every division, the telomere at the end of the DNA shortens a bit more. After a certain number of divisions, the telomeres are exhausted and the cell becomes senescent, or dead. This limit is known as the Hayflick limit, named after the researcher Leonard Hayflick, who discovered in 1961 that cells had a maximum limit to the number of times they can divide before they die. For most cells, the Hayflick limit is forty to sixty divisions before it dies.* After cell death, the cell debris is cleaned up to make room for new, healthy cells.

As people age, their telomeres shorten and the Hayflick limit decreases, meaning older people no longer experience the longer cell life and healthy cell division of their youth. Instead, their cells die off more quickly, becoming loaded down with junk DNA and mutations with every division. In some cases, these half-dead cells remain as a kind of zombie cell, not really

---

* The Embryo Project Encyclopedia. The Hayflick limit. https://embryo.asu.edu/pages/hayflick-limit.

functioning but excreting inflammatory and dangerous chemicals—or even worse mutating into pre-cancerous or cancerous cells!

After discovering the role of telomeres in the cell lifecycle, researchers found that some kinds of cells need to live longer because of their unique function. This includes sperm cells, white blood cells, and stem cells.* In these cells, an enzyme called telomerase actually adds length to the telomere, allowing the cells to divide more than regular cells and experience a longer functional lifespan. Cancer cells, which are defined by unregulated division and deadly growth, have a defective telomerase system that makes them immortal.

According to the telomere theory of aging, if we could figure out a way to preserve or even lengthen the telomeres on healthy cells, those cells would gain extra divisions and contribute to the health of that organ or tissue. The key, however, is finding a way to do this without creating cancerous cells that never die and while also somehow still limiting DNA mutations and defects within the dividing cells.

Fortunately, this is one of the areas that we as integrative and regenerative medicine practitioners have seen grow in leaps and bounds in the last ten years. We understand cells, free radicals, telomeres, and DNA better than ever. We know that wonderful therapies, such as ozone, glutathione, NAD, NAD+, micronutrient IVs, hormone optimizing, stem cell and exosome therapies, hyperbaric oxygen, and infrared are all readily available, safe, and effective ways to increase telomerase, slow down telomere shortening, improve mitochondria function, and inhibit and reverse the aging process!

Environmental Toxins and Stress

Finally, aging is affected by two more external factors: environmental toxins and stress. While both of these contribute to inflammation, they also cause damage that goes beyond inflammation.

A good example of how environmental toxins affect human health is breast cancer. According to the highly respected Susan G. Komen Foundation, which advocates for women and is working to help end breast cancer, there has been a dramatic increase in breast cancer over the past

---

* Razgonova MP, Zakharenko AM, Golokhvast KS, et al. Telomerase and telomeres in aging theory and chronographic aging theory (Review). *Mol Med Rep.* 2020;22(3):1679-1694. doi:10.3892/mmr.2020.11274.

thirty years. This increase has coincided with an increase in exposure to environmental toxins including DDT (now banned, but still present in water and food), bisphenol A (BPA) found in plastic products, polycyclic aromatic hydrocarbons (PAHs), parabens, PCBs, phthalates, heavy metals, pesticides, herbicides, arsenic, lead, and dioxins.*

These are all known carcinogens that in some cases can imitate the effects of estrogen in the body and may be contributing to breast cancer in vulnerable women. Dozens of animal studies have confirmed that exposure to toxins increases breast cancer risk, but there remains some question about the effect they have in humans. The confusion isn't centered on whether the chemicals are dangerous—we know they are—but exactly how much effect they have. It turns out it's almost impossible to measure the effect of any one isolated environmental factor in human health, thanks to the incredible diversity of the way people live and even our own biology. Population studies attempting to prove that low-level, chronic exposure to dioxin contributes to all types of cancer, for example, have to find a way to control for individual diet, genetics, exposure to other chemicals, socioeconomic status, exercise status, comorbidities, and a galaxy of other influences before they can isolate the role dioxin might play in cancer formation.

Not only is this an almost impossible task, it's a slow one. Proving that environmental toxins are dangerous enough to actually regulate them takes years of study and requires overcoming fierce industry opposition in most cases. Even as underfunded researchers work to prove that our increasing exposure to toxins is helping kill us, rich industries like the petrochemical industry push back with their own studies and lobby government agencies.

All this time, more and more of these chemicals are pushed into the environment, multiplying the toxic stress that we are surrounded by twenty-four hours a day, seven days a week. In effect, we are all involuntary subjects in the largest public health experiment in human history, whether we want to be or not. In too many cases, by the time we finally have enough information to act, the damage is already done.

Even if we are sometimes challenged to prove the connection between individual toxins and health problems, we can step back and look at what's happening across society. Autoimmune disorders like asthma and allergies are skyrocketing, along with serious respiratory illnesses like COPD. Rates of autism are shooting up, with murky causes. Certain cancers are becoming more common, including breast and prostate, which are both

---

* The Susan G. Komen Foundation. Environmental chemicals and breast cancer risk. https://blog.komen.org/blog/komen-perspectives-environmental-chemicals-and-breast-cancer-risk/

hormone-mediated. Female reproductive cycles are changing in permanent ways that we don't fully understand, including the much earlier onset of puberty. Infertility is rising. Incidences of neurological disorders and dementia are rising.

All of this can't be a coincidence—and there's almost no other explanation that makes sense except that we are living in an increasingly toxic world that bombards our DNA daily, causing mutations that accumulate and degrade our health.

Finally, there's the elephant in the room: stress. We all know what stress is, and it's common to think we have the highest amounts of it compared to others. But stress is literally a killer. We can no longer let stress ruin our lives. Even if some stress is inevitable, we can help people's bodies better adapt and compensate for their stress levels. We work with our patients to ensure that their lifestyles are no longer an acceptable scapegoat for poor health and instead help them focus on preventing long-term stress from aging their bodies any faster.

The picture that emerges in anti-aging medicine is both depressing and hopeful. It's challenging because of the forces arrayed against us. In the beginning of the book, I noted that, for the first time in more than a century, life expectancy in the United States declined in the opening decades of the 21st century. This was thanks to diseases of despair, including alcoholism, and suicide—but it's also a symptom of the world we have created. We are immersed in an environment that seems designed to make us sick and age faster. And who's to blame? Who would possibly benefit from this situation? The answer is depressingly obvious. Corporate food interests. Pharmaceutical companies. A bloated and expensive medical industry. Even chemical and petrochemical companies get in on the act of profiting from our disease. It can feel overwhelming.

But there is hope, too, and that's one of my central messages. As an individual, there may not be much you or I can do about the presence of toxins in the environment or change the food industry—but there's a lot each of us can do about our own health. And today, we know more than we ever have about how to preserve health and life. There's so much high-quality information out there, it's only a matter of teaching patients how to recognize information they can trust and give them the tools to create a healthy lifestyle plan that will improve their daily lives and give them more years of high-quality time. Age is just a number, but the number on your driver's license is not necessarily the age you should live your life by. At our practice, we help people assess, interpret, and give you the tools necessary to help impede and reverse the aging process. Gone are the days of thinking we can live until only seventy or eighty; people are now living into their hundreds. To me, that's only worth doing if you can maintain the quality and functionality of life to make those elder years worth living the way you desire.

Chapter 13

What Society Gets Wrong About Aging

"Age is an issue of mind over matter. If you don't mind, it doesn't matter."

—**Mark Twain**

In the last chapter, I discussed the factors that drive real aging. These are the targets of true anti-aging medicine, and I believe it's entirely possible that thanks to anti-aging medicine, we'll see the first 130-year-old human in the next generation. Despite the many challenges we currently face, I believe we're on the brink of an explosion in human life span. Better yet, I believe we'll be adding "good" years to our lives as people learn to live deep into their old age with a higher quality of life.

But here's an interesting thing: unless you subscribe to certain media outlets, or seek it out, you'd never know this is true from our mainstream health media. Sure, a big magazine might run a feature on anti-aging medicine occasionally, or *The New York Times* will report on some breakthrough, but there's very little focus on the actual advances that may soon change the way humans relate to and think about aging. And guess what? It should not take a catchy headline or trendy celebrity secret to motivate you to listen and learn and get the critical knowledge it takes to maximize longevity and quality of life.

Yet instead of learning about the revolution in anti-aging medicine, what do we get? A cultural, relentless focus on physical appearances and looks. Let's face it: sex sells. The media, along with social media, has drastically changed the way we all look at ourselves and what we consider to be aging. We are subjected to an endless stream of marketing pitches to restore youthful looks, erase wrinkles, and feel younger—and not all of it is effective or even honest. Pharmaceutical companies push pills that promise to restore youthful sex drive and hair growth. And I'm sorry to say, many alternative health practitioners and supplement companies market products, goods, therapies, and potions as fountains of youth that can fix any issue, often using the same highly deceptive language as the snake-oil salesmen of older times. I hate to generalize, because there are wonderful organizations and companies that do amazing things, but too many are looking to sell the "quick fix" rather than focusing on what we all know impacts aging the most.

The result is that we are confused. We've been conditioned to focus on the exterior signs of youth when aging is really an internal process. Aging is a biological and chemical-physiologic process that starts at the cellular level and is impacted by a broad spectrum of factors ranging from genetics to environment to lifestyle choices and the age-related degenerative processes that our bodies go through over time. Aging doesn't happen from the outside skin or receding hairline—aging starts from the inside at the cellular level and works outward. The irony of this is that many of the signs that we associate with aging—like hair loss and wrinkling—may have literally nothing to do with aging at all but are just genetic traits that are passed down through families.

At the same time, we're subjected to intensive youth marketing, we're also bombarded with products and messaging for things that are literally killing us. I'm talking about unhealthy food, alcohol, and toxic products. Just looking at alcohol alone, according to *Business Insider*, alcohol companies spend a little under half a billion dollars every year advertising their wares.* Further, much of this is aimed at teens and younger adults. The idea is to hook new drinkers on particular brands and drinks as early as possible and create lifelong customers. The ill-health effects of this are obvious—alcohol is a known toxin that may result in broken families, tens of thousands of deaths every year, rampant addiction, and social misery.

---

* American Addiction Centers. Rules & regulations about marketing alcohol. https://www.alcohol.org/laws/marketing-to-the-public/

Since we're on the topic of powerful media influences and strategic marketing, what about the biggest way these media outlets really kill us without even trying? The media is supposed to inform us, but what does it really do? In truth, with gotcha headlines and bad reporting, the media creates confusion and sends mixed messages, driving stress levels through the roof and influencing the way you make health decisions. We are subtly told we are not working hard enough or long enough, or that we need to make more money, have a certain status, drive a certain car, or live in a certain zip code. This constant messaging affects our cognitive expectations, which affects our neurotransmitters, and then what do you think happens? Our ability to make positive health decisions is compromised and mass numbers of people are confused as the mass media changes the way we act, think, and live. The tragedy is that, since we know mass media has the ability to change behavior, we are passing up the opportunity to encourage better health and spread good information. Instead, beset on all sides by bad information, we are encouraged to make decisions that kill us.*

In addition to all of this media pressure, we are short on sleep, eating too much, not getting enough exercise, and generally living like there is no tomorrow, much less another forty or fifty years of potentially healthy lifespan.

So, this is my message to patients: STOP. It's time to get off the hamster wheel of disease and destruction and misguided ways of thinking that surround us. It's time to make better choices to slow the aging process and do our part to inhibit or slow the aging process. We have the information, and we know what works. We've studied enough long-lived populations, like the Japanese in Okinawa or villagers in Italy who live on seasonal produce and lean protein, to know that a certain lifestyle is definitely linked to less disease and better quality of life. And we've unlocked the relatively simple formula that makes it possible:

- Healthy balanced diet
- Good sleep, minimizing stress
- Strong social connections
- Plenty of exercise, even into old age

While it's easy to get lost in confusing marketing messages or detailed arguments about what is optimal, the general contours of a healthy lifestyle

---

* https://www.tandfonline.com/doi/abs/10.1080/01639360802265863.

are well known and available to anyone. You don't need a catchy headline or a breaking news medical report to tell you these things.

If we don't find a way to break out of this cycle or change our mindset as individuals and as a society, the consequences are also well known. In 2020, the world was under assault from the coronavirus. By the time the virus will have been fully under control, it will likely have been linked and associated with the death or influencing of almost a million Americans. While this is a great tragedy, it's also a little bit of an anomaly in our modern world. Today, unlike previous centuries, our greatest threat doesn't come from viruses or deadly bacteria. Instead, our biggest dangers are the so-called lifestyle diseases that are linked to our own behaviors and lifestyles. Sometimes called "diseases of aging," this rogues' gallery of diseases includes the biggest killers in America today: heart disease, cancer, diabetes, liver disease, kidney disease, and more recently, autoimmune disorders.

The tragedy of focusing on cosmetic signs of aging is that it distracts us from the more urgent work of controlling these diseases of aging, especially the ones that are largely preventable through better, more informed decision-making. And once again, we must recognize the tactics of mass media and social media platforms that use youth, vitality, and anti-aging campaigns to distract us from understanding how our bodies work and what parameters control aging.

Consider the effect this has on just heart disease. According to the Centers for Disease Control and Prevention, as many as 200,000 deaths from heart disease are preventable every year. More than half of these occur in people under sixty-five years of age.* Overall, the CDC estimates that 15 percent of all cancer deaths, 30 percent of heart disease deaths, 36 percent of deaths caused by lung disease, and 28 percent of all stroke deaths are preventable.†

Think about this. Literally hundreds of thousands of Americans are dying every year from choices they are making thanks to subtle pressure from mass media. Many millions more are not being helped because their healthcare practitioners don't have the time or patience to discuss easy-to-implement lifestyle changes that can literally safe their lives. Too many people are carrying a terrible burden of disease, contributing to the healthcare debt of this country, unable to work, spending tens of thousands of

---

* Centers for Disease Control & Prevention. Preventable deaths from heart disease and stroke. https://www.cdc.gov/vitalsigns/heartdisease-stroke/index.html.

† Centers for Disease Control & Prevention. CDC estimates preventable deaths from 5 leading causes. https://www.cdc.gov/media/releases/2016/p1117-preventable-deaths.html.

dollars on treatments, and suffering from greatly reduced quality of life. It must stop!

It doesn't have to be this way. As a healthcare provider, I know we can do better, and it begins with helping patients understand how to find a healthy balance in their lives. This doesn't mean prescribing extreme diets of exclusion, like zero-carb diets or calorie restriction, or asking patients to launch exercise programs that may be impossible for them to maintain. I am always a realist with my patients, and I don't think it is fair to expect people to implement these turnarounds overnight. It sets them up for failure. A more reasonable and modest, gradual approach based on lifestyle education is the key to success, which is why it is of upmost importance to start young and stay ahead of the disease curve! Patients need accurate information they can use to create a diet that's right for their unique physiology, get enough exercise to stay strong and flexible, and work with their medical team to monitor their changing bodies and catch problems early, before they develop into serious conditions.

I know this is possible, because I've worked with thousands of patients in our clinics to turn their lives around. I've seen patients with heart disease transform their lives to the point where they no longer need prescription heart medications. I've worked with people to design diets they can actually live with, that let them eat the things they like while still sticking to mostly healthy foods that nourish their bodies. And we've encouraged people to take up exercise programs that fit their lifestyles, even if that just means taking a brisk walk a few times a week. And the results of this are so encouraging—these patients enjoy a healthy glow from within, enjoying a more enduring health than any cosmetic procedure could possibly give them.

The key is understanding why our bodies age, how our bodies age, and understanding the factors that people can control to mitigate the long-term complications of our modern lifestyle. We cannot continue to fall victim to these media-created perceptions of aging and what is healthy and unhealthy. We must avoid the false notions presented by mainstream media and their corporate allies and not succumb to their time-tested marketing campaigns and tactics. Instead, as healthcare practitioners, we need to show patients they have the knowledge and the resources to take their health into their own hands.

Chapter 14

Anti-Aging
Medicine

"The skilful doctor treats those who are well but the inferior doctor treats those who are ill."

—Ch'in Yueh-jen

Anti-aging medicine is one of the most exciting branches in medicine today—but ironically, I'm not a big fan of the phrase "anti-aging" when it comes to medicine. As valuable as this new branch of research and clinical practice is, the words "anti-aging" don't really capture what we're trying to do. When you hear the phrase "anti-aging" medicine, what pops into your head? Most people would say they think about Botox and beauty treatments, right? For most of us, aging is associated with only our exteriors, which is why medical practices that call themselves "anti-aging" practices are not really doing what we are talking about. In fact, we're not fighting "aging," but instead trying to slow down or even reverse degenerative diseases that affect the aging process and rob people of their quality of life and time on this planet. I prefer to think of our scope of medicine as regenerative medicine, and it really forms the core of everything we're doing in our clinics.

When it comes to regenerative medicine and anti-aging programs, I like to describe a three-legged stool. The legs include:

- Lifestyle changes (the things you can control and influence)
- Regenerative medicine (the tools we can provide to support the other two)
- DNA health (the way your body is programmed to operate)

In this chapter, we'll take a closer look at each of these and how they can work together in a successful integrative medicine approach to support patients as they regain control over their own health.

Lifestyle Changes

This point can't be emphasized or repeated enough: a healthy lifestyle is the foundation of longevity and optimal health. What would you expect to happen to a Lamborghini if you put in regular unleaded fuel, never changed the air filters, and ran the engine twenty-four hours a day, seven days a week? How long until the car stops working? There's overwhelming evidence that a person who eats a healthy diet, gets adequate exercise, and takes active steps to reduce stress, get enough sleep, and manage their own health is a person who will live a longer, healthier life. We can see this in real life among the long-lived, healthy populations of people in the Blue Zones.*

People in Blue Zones aren't genetically superior or have access to some secret Fountain of Youth that the rest of us don't have. In reality, for a variety of reasons having to do with culture, history, and geography, people in these diverse regions simply live healthier lives, with a greater focus on strong social connections, healthier diets with an emphasis on fresh produce, lots of exercise, and a stronger spiritual connection.

Even if you don't live in a Blue Zone, there are plenty of lessons here for the rest of us. First and most importantly, they show the value of moderation. People who live in Blue Zones aren't pursuing exotic diets or unusual longevity eating programs. While I have nothing against these programs if they work for patients, the fact is that most people don't want to follow strict, exclusionary diets for the long term. Also, there's no single diet that I can recommend that would work for everyone. As we've discussed, everybody is different. What works for me may not work for you. Some people

---

* Wikipedia. Blue Zones. https://en.wikipedia.org/wiki/Blue_Zone.

Dr. Daly's Advice: Start with the Gut

My colleague Rosemary Daly, DO, has some good advice for where to start when it comes to improving health: the gut.

"We can all start by doing simple things to promote digestive health: change our diets and allow the body to heal and eliminate toxins in a natural way," she says.

This means eating lots of organic leafy greens and fermented vegetables, plus unprocessed meat and cultured dairy products, while cutting out the gluten, reducing stress, and reducing alcohol and caffeine.

"This doesn't mean ignoring your symptoms," she says. "You need to explain symptoms to your doctor and certain tests may be necessary. But if your physicians rule out underlying metabolic disease, there's no reason not to start re-building your gut health."

---

do better with higher carbohydrate intake, while others can't eat too many carbs without unpleasant side effects.

So, what does lifestyle moderation look like when it comes to successful anti-aging? Not surprisingly, it begins with good data. I recommend all patients start with food sensitivity testing so they can begin to understand how food interacts with their unique biology. After that, we have a variety of tools we can use to encourage better diet:

- *Blood chemistry testing*: This can help identify deficiencies in micronutrients or other issues, such as excess systemic inflammation, that may be linked to diet.

- *Blood typing*: Blood type can be closely linked to food sensitivity and dietary needs.

- *Neurotransmitter testing*: This one surprises many people, who think only of neurotransmitters in the brain. Actually, about 80 percent of our neurotransmitters are produced in the gut and are intimately linked to gut function, mood, and overall health. This connection is sometimes called the "gut/brain," and it's critical to health.

Once a baseline is established, we can track these markers to see how a person's body is interacting with and responding to the food they eat. It's also crucial that patients learn how to pay attention to their own bodies. If someone gets bad gas or pain after eating a certain food, that's a signal that this particular food doesn't agree with their biology. This goes far beyond the bloated, sick feeling people often report after eating too much garbage food or junk food. Many people may react to a food for years and try to ignore it (or they don't even manifest the damage it is causing), until they learn this food really doesn't agree with them. Part of my job is giving my patients the tools and education to recognize this.

I also strongly believe in using dietary supplements to "fill the gaps" in your diet. While a comprehensive, custom supplementation program can only be designed after extensive blood testing for individual patients, we focus on the "core four" supplements in our practice. These include:

- *Coenzyme Q10 with PQQ*: This combination has been shown to increase the bioavailability of coenzyme Q10, which is linked to improved heart health and mitochondrial function.

- *Vitamin D3/K2*: Vitamin D is actually a pro-hormone that supports a healthy immune system and has many biological effects. Most people are at least slightly deficient in vitamin D.

- *Omega-3 fatty acid*: These fatty acids, found in cold-water fish, support healthy brain function and heart function, as well as improved bone function through reduced inflammation. Most people don't get enough omega-3 fatty acids, so supplementation is vital.

- *Hormonal support*: This may be the single most important thing aging people can do for themselves. As we age, our hormone levels drop dramatically, with dire effects for our health. Hormonal support can erase many of the damaging aspects of aging, providing that the hormone support program is carefully designed and managed.

This basic package is a great place to start for overall support, but most aging people also benefit from additional supplement support, especially to help control chronic inflammation. Additional supplement programs should be based on the results of blood testing and the patient's history.

About Exercise

Imagine if there was a single prescription that could dramatically reduce the risk of heart disease and stroke, diabetes, obesity, osteoporosis, and depression, while also extending years of quality of life. Such a prescription would be the biggest breakthrough in medicine since antibiotics and vaccines were developed and represent a major breakthrough in human health.

You can probably guess where I'm going with this, but such a prescription already exists: exercise.

Getting adequate weight-bearing exercise is one of the healthiest things any person can do for themselves. It affects everything from insulin levels to mood. Exercise has been shown to help reduce cholesterol, control blood pressure, aid in healthy weight loss, protect bones, and help ward off the frailty that affects so many aging people. Current recommendations for exercise include:

- Children and adolescents (6 to 17 years): 60 minutes of moderate-to-vigorous physical activity every day.

- Adults (18 to 64 years): A minimum of 150 minutes of moderate intensity activity a week.

- Older adults (65 years and older): A minimum of moderate intensity activity every week, plus balancing exercises.*

Unfortunately, we're nowhere near getting enough physical activity as a society. According to the National Health and Nutrition Examination Study (NHANES) that looked at the exercise habits of more than fifty thousand people, sedentary behavior increased among all age groups between 2001 and 2016. Overall, researchers found that adults and teenagers spend an astonishing 8.2 hours in front of screens or sitting every day.†

Among healthcare providers, these results are really no surprise—how often do we tell patients they need to get more exercise and eat better, even when it's unlikely the message will actually change behavior? This conundrum is really at the heart of my whole approach to practicing medicine. We can tell people all day what they "should" be doing, but until patients have internalized the information, really understand it, and believe it, there's little chance they'll act on it. Already, patients are bombarded with messages every day to get more exercise, but change comes from within, not from any well-meaning advice from a doctor or healthcare provider.

---

* Centers for Disease Control and Prevention. Physical activity recommendations for different age groups. https://www.cdc.gov/physicalactivity/basics/age-chart.html

† Trends in sedentary behavior among the US population, 2001-2016. JAMA 2019;321:1587-1597.

So, the question becomes: how can we help patients incorporate exercise into their lives?

First, we have to honestly address the messaging surrounding exercise in this country. Earlier, we examined how marketing messages around healthcare focus on the external and aesthetic. Nowhere is this more prevalent than in the cultural messaging surrounding exercise. Every year, billions of dollars are spent by gyms, exercise equipment companies, and supplement companies selling people on the "benefits" of exercise. And what are those benefits in most cases? Six-pack abs. Sex appeal. Bulging muscles. Models, typically in their twenties, are shown dripping with sweat while grunting under piles of weights, performing intimidating CrossFit routines or sprinting up mountainsides.

This is *not* the message we should be sending when we talk about exercise. Exercise does have powerful aesthetic benefits, but they are secondary to what really matters when it comes to keeping fit. Moreover, focusing on that type of messaging can be discouraging for patients who are older or struggling with excess weight. Far from inspiring, unattainable perfection can discourage people from even starting to exercise.

Instead, just as with diet, I like to focus on making exercise achievable and realistic for every patient. For some patients, this might mean punishing exercise regimens with weights or CrossFit, but even in those cases, I don't think this is a viable long-term approach. The human body wasn't built to withstand punishment for years on end. In our clinics, I've worked with plenty of current and former professional athletes, including football players, whose bodies are decades older than their chronological age and suffering from joint issues and physical problems.

When it comes to talking to patients about exercise, I always emphasize a few points:

- Exercise should not only address strength through weight-bearing exercises, but also flexibility. This is especially important for older adults, who are at risk of fractures from falling.

- You should enjoy exercise! Find something you like to do and try to work it into your daily activities. Exercise can include things like walking briskly along the beach, dancing, or gardening. This is called functional movement, and it can be and should be the foundation of a healthy lifestyle.

- Weight-bearing exercise is important as you age, but this doesn't mean you're in the gym seven days a week doing deadlifts. Even

a small amount of weight is enough for most people to achieve
the benefits.

• It's never too late! There's no age at which it's too late to start
  exercising, and the benefits of exercise are open to all adults.
  If you have a pre-existing health condition, however, it's very
  important to work with a healthcare provider and/or qualified
  trainer to design an exercise program that is safe.

Beyond these simple guidelines, I don't advise any particular program. Whatever form exercise takes, it's all good when it comes to helping
patients live longer, healthier, and happier lives.

Sleep and Stress

As important as diet and exercise are, they aren't the only lifestyle factors
that have a direct effect on both the length and quality of life. Getting adequate sleep and finding ways to reduce or manage stress are also directly
related to disease risk and overall mortality. These two areas of life may be
the most influential in maintaining homeostasis and overall quality, functionality, and duration of life. Ironically, these two areas that may contribute the most to our lifespan are two of the parameters we have the strongest
influence over.

When it comes to sleep, my message is that quantity of sleep isn't the
most important factor. Just like almost everything else when it comes to
health, different people have different sleep needs. Some people do just fine
on five hours of sleep a night, while others feel exhausted after eight hours
of sleep. Instead of worrying about how many hours we're lying in bed,
we should be paying attention to getting high-quality sleep. At the most
basic level, this means practicing good sleep hygiene. When it's bedtime,
the room should be dark and comfortable, without televisions, phones, or
other sources of blue light that affect sleep quality. Additionally, for people
who do consume alcohol, drinking right before bedtime may feel relaxing,
but it actually reduces the quality of sleep.

Getting quality sleep is especially important for shift workers or people who maintain unusual hours, including firefighters, police, and other
professions. Among this group, the lack of a predictable circadian rhythm
wreaks havoc with their adrenal glands, which further complicates sleep.
For this group, supportive means are often necessary to help maintain
homeostasis and ensure their bodies are entering into deep REM sleep.

How can we expect our bodies to repair, heal, and regenerate if we never give our body the ability to turn off and recoup?

Finally, there's stress. We live in a stressful society and, especially during the COVID-19 pandemic, a stressful time. For many, many of us, there's really no easy way to minimize stress, so it can feel defeating to simply announce that patients have to "reduce stress." When people are worried about their relatives, their livelihoods, and the rapid pace of technology and cultural change, telling someone to cut their stress down can seem like empty words. Sometimes I have to wonder: is this stressful lifestyle really necessary? Or is it driven by mass media outlets?

Whatever the answer, stress can also be a relative thing, as some people do not cope with stress as well as others, and varying levels of stress impact people in different ways. We must recognize that stress is a part of our lives no matter what we do, and our goal is not to set unrealistic expectations of getting rid of stress but rather helping our bodies minimize the negative impacts of stress. Better yet, how can we help or support our body's ability to compensate and adapt to stress? Those are the questions we need to be asking ourselves and our practitioners.

There's no question stress contributes to health problems and worsens quality of life. So, what can we do about it? The first step is often to take a full hormone panel and look for signs of adrenal dysfunction and hormone imbalance, then taking steps to improve and optimize any underlying imbalances. The same applies for neurotransmitters: any imbalances in neurotransmitters should be addressed to help improve mood and restore homeostasis. After that, many of the same tools we recommend elsewhere are important. Exercise can help reduce stress by stimulating the natural production of the feel-good chemical's dopamine and serotonin. Meditation also works, if people are interested and willing to learn how. Believe me, learning how to properly mediate makes all the difference in the world. Social connections are vital too, so as much as possible, we should be socializing with loved ones and friends, even if it's over videoconference. Social interaction releases large amounts of the hormone oxytocin which can help reduce adrenal production of cortisol, balance out sex and thyroid hormones, and instill a calm and stable mood. Cut down on screen time and avoid stressful inputs, including the news (the largest influencer of stress for many people).

We teach our patients to learn to recognize the first signs of increased stress—changes in breathing patterns like holding breath, physical symptoms like tinnitus, extra night snacking, increased alcohol consumption—and provide support to help them make better choices.

Promoting Healthy DNA

Over the past few decades, our understanding of DNA and its role in day-to-day health has increased exponentially. In earlier decades, there was a perception that DNA helped "code" our basic traits, like hair and eye color and disease risk, but its effect on day-to-day health wasn't understood as well. Instead, we viewed DNA more like a master switch that helped determine who we were and assumed that genetic change—in the form of mutations—was a slow-moving process.

It turns out this simplistic view of genetic mutability and inheritance was missing a few important elements. In reality, genetic expression can change rapidly, even over the course of a single life, and insults to DNA can have a profound effect on an individual's health.

We know this, in part, thanks to the science of epigenetics. The epigenome is a series of chemical "switches" that wraps around the main DNA code. In the simplest terms, the epigenome can control whether a gene is expressed, or whether it's expressed fully or partially.* Think of the epigenome as the keyboard that controls the central "computer" of DNA, and like a keyboard, the epigenome is much more sensitive to external input than the DNA itself. Epigenetic injuries, caused by inflammation, disease, toxins, or other causes, can contribute to sickness by causing damage to DNA. Over time, as DNA defects accumulate, the overall risk of contracting a disease like cancer significantly increases.

So, what can we do to support a healthy genome and slow the rate of epigenetic injury and the accumulation of dangerous DNA defects? First, it's important to understand that DNA is not destiny. A family history of heart disease or cancer does not mean you are going to get heart disease and cancer. When you consider the ability of the epigenome to affect genetic expression from decade to decade, it means we have much greater control over our immediate genetic history than many people think.

Second, there are concrete steps we can take to protect our epigenome and, therefore, our DNA. Not surprisingly, many of these will look familiar:

- *Eat a healthy diet.* Foods that are overcooked or burned, heavily processed, and full of preservatives have been shown to cause direct damage to the epigenome. This means limiting

---

* Ganesan, A., Arimondo, P.B., Rots, M.G. et al. The timeline of epigenetic drug discovery: from reality to dreams. *Clin Epigenet* 11, 174 (2019). https://doi.org/10.1186/s13148-019-0776-0.

dangerous foods like cured deli meats and smoked foods like barbecue. Similarly, getting enough folic acid is key, because folic acid provides the building blocks for DNA synthesis and is critical to a process called methylation that, when disturbed, can damage DNA.

- *Maintain a healthy gut biome.* The gut biome interacts with the epigenome, either positively or negatively. A healthy gut biome will supply the building blocks of DNA and the neurotransmitters needed to ensure healthy cell replication.

- *Get good sleep.* When we sleep, our bodies conduct vital "housekeeping" processes, like flushing away damaged and aging cells. Lack of high-quality sleep, especially as we age, reduces our ability to conduct this genetic housekeeping and can increase the risk of DNA damage.

- *Control stress.* Stress activates hormone feedback loops that flood the body with adrenaline and other chemicals. In short bursts, this poses no threat to the DNA, but over time, chronic stress can contribute to epigenetic damage.*

Regenerative Medicine

The final leg of my three-legged anti-aging stool is regenerative medicine. While the first two legs of the stool are largely in patients' hands, as long as they are empowered to make good choices, this final element is where qualified healthcare practitioners come in. Regenerative medicine is defined as the effort to slow or reverse disease processes. Unlike more traditional allopathic medicine, which is often aimed at alleviating symptoms and ignoring the underlying disease process, regenerative medicine goes another level deeper to attack the disease process itself.

This is really the heart of our medical approach. Regenerative medicine offers a full quiver of tools that work together to promote health from the cellular and microscopic level. We've discussed many of them throughout the book already, but I'll give a high-level overview of the ones we turn to most in our clinic. As we're looking at these, however, it's vital to understand two key points.

---

* Ferguson, Bradley S. *Nutritional Epigenetics.* Academic Press; 2019.

First, none of these are magic cure-alls. If there's one critical message to take away from this book, it's that every person is unique, with distinct needs and biology. Good medicine takes the time to understand each patient and design therapeutic programs that work for them. We don't prescribe statins to every patient who walks in the door, because not every patient with elevated cholesterol needs statin medication. Instead, we use testing and extensive histories to create a deep understanding of everything going on, then address areas of concern with customized programs.

Second, none of these are meant to work alone. A comprehensive anti-aging program isn't built on just bioidentical hormone replacement, or just infusion therapy, or just anti-inflammatory diets. Once we've gained a deep understanding of individual patients, the goal is to create a program uniquely suited for that patient and communicate it in a way that fully educates and informs the patient both about what we're trying to do and what they can do to support their own health.

With this said, here are some of the therapeutic tools we frequently utilize to help patients turn back the clock on aging and disease.

Hormone Optimization

Hormone optimization is one of the most powerful anti-aging therapeutic approaches available today. In healthy younger people, hormone levels are naturally balanced, regulating growth, development, sex drive, mood, metabolism, and dozens of other biological functions. As we age, however, hormone levels begin to decline and become imbalanced, leading to both obvious symptoms (like hair loss, menopause, and fat accumulation) and not-so-obvious symptoms like fatigue, depression, and a compromised immune system.

Hormone optimization is highly personalized and depends on thorough and ongoing testing to establish a baseline and then monitor the therapy. Hormones we can adjust include sex hormones like estrogen, progesterone, testosterone, and DHEA, as well as thyroid hormones and other hormones. A balanced, youthful hormone system can have a profound impact on both quality of life and disease risk, with reductions in risk for certain cancers, heart attack, and stroke. The key to success with hormone optimization is balance—hormones all work together; one dysfunction in one hormone can easily have a cascade effect throughout the endocrine system.

It's important to note, however, that education is a critical part of hormone therapy. Thanks to the widespread use of synthetic hormones among menopausal women, which was shown to increase the risk of breast cancer, many aging women believe they will get breast cancer if they start using bioidentical hormones. Similarly, many men hear "testosterone" and immediately think they are taking anabolic steroids. In reality, a well-designed hormone program uses the smallest effective dose of the highest-quality hormones available to re-establish youthful levels and actually protect patients from diseases including prostate and breast cancer, as well as reduce stroke and heart attack risk.

Micronutrient Infusion Therapy

This is one of the most exciting areas of medicine to me. Infusion therapy is cutting-edge medicine that addresses some of the most common underlying issues associated with aging, including declining gut function. In today's advanced and obesogenic society, we need to question the integrity and quality of food and vitamins, plus take into account our stress levels and environment and how they affect gut function and absorption of vitamins, minerals, nutrients, and critical amino acids.

Micronutrient therapy is the best way to ensure that our bodies not only receive but also maintain and store the highest concentrations of critical compounds. With micronutrient IV therapy, we have the ability to bypass the body's digestive and filtration systems and directly provide key substances in the most bioavailable form. By delivering infusions directly into the bloodstream, nutrients can circulate into our tissues without wasting time and energy metabolizing anything. Our IV therapies allow our team to customize and bring unique therapy offerings to each individual patient.

Ozone Therapy

We all know the power of oxygen—it gives life. Ozone therapy delivers an extra oxygen molecule (instead of normal O2, ozone is O3), which allows the highly concentrated molecule to diffuse through the body and into tissues. Oxygen is arguably the most important element in the body, as it affects every cell function, including energy production, detoxification, and respiration. By super-charging the body with oxygen, ozone therapy is anti-viral, anti-bacterial, anti-fungal, anti-parasitic, anti-inflammatory, immunomodulating, cancer-inhibiting, and much more. Ozone therapy not only helps slow or reverse disease and degeneration, it also has the ability to stimulate stem cells, produce more effective mitochondria, detoxify the body, and lengthen telomeres.*

Neurotransmitter Therapy

Neurotransmitter therapy is a fast-developing area of anti-aging medicine with profound implications for overall health. Most neurotransmitters are actually produced in the gut, where they can help regulate everything from metabolism to mood. When we're testing neurotransmitters levels, we are actually measuring underlying gut health as well as brain health.

Combined with specific GI testing for enzymes, waste products, and indicators of digestive function, we can create a robust program of gut support and restoration using neurotransmitters, probiotics, prebiotics, and digestive enzymes. The result is improved digestion and immune system health, better mood, and protection from disease.

Stem Cell and Exosome Therapies

This is another area of medicine that has recently exploded, for good and not-so-good reasons. This scope of practice in regenerative medicine has been controversial for the last ten to twenty-five years. Today, it's unfortunately one of the most scrutinized area of regenerative medicine. I say "unfortunate" because this therapy is arguably the most effective and non-invasive way to help regenerate damage to our bodies.

Despite what you may think, stem cell therapies are not new. In fact, bone marrow–derived cell procedures date back to the 1970s. However, through a combination of poor education and unscrupulous healthcare practitioners looking to turn a quick buck, stem cell therapy has become a questionable form of regenerative therapy.

There are two different forms of regenerative stem cell therapies:

- Autologous, meaning stem cells derived from your body
- Allogenic, or stem cells harvested from donor tissues

---

* https://www.lifeworkswellnesscenter.com/ozone-therapy/how-does-ozone-therapy-work.html.

As we age, stem cells become less effective and can even become dormant or non-functioning. As this happens, more stem cells lose the ability to regenerate and mend damaged parts of our bodies, which results in inflammation, disease, and death. Stem cell therapy addresses this by providing a source of new stem cells to aging bodies. As stem cell therapy has advanced, we have become proficient at using these stem cell therapies to help regenerate tissues in all of our major organ systems including: orthopedic and sports injuries, chronic inflammatory conditions, autoimmune conditions, neurodegenerative conditions, and even as a preventative health measure.

And despite what you may have heard, stem cell and exosome therapies are not illegal in the U.S.!

As the science and research into stem cell therapies continues to advance, we are learning about new and exciting "cellular" therapies such as exosome therapy, which uses a stem cell byproduct to signal or attract stem cells to damaged tissues. Think of exosomes as similar to a road flare—they let your body know where help is needed. These incredibly tiny particles may be even more powerful than mesenchymal stem cells, as a fire truck does you no good if you can't find the fire!

Both of these cellular regenerative therapies are critical if your goal is slowing down or reversing the aging process and a staple in my practices.*

---

* https://www.ncbi.nlm.nih.gov/pmc/articles/PMC4823383/.

Chapter 15

The Future Is Now

Biohacking (N): The art and science of changing the environment around you and inside you, so you have more control over your own biology.

We live in a remarkable age. On the one hand, we are dealing with tremendous challenges in our healthcare system. Unique among industrialized nations, our healthcare system shifts the burden of paying for care onto citizens. The result is a wildly expensive system that leaves us all one accident or diagnosis away from bankruptcy and financial ruin. Simultaneously, corporate and moneyed interests have used their billions to purchase tremendous influence, meaning that we prioritize the financial concerns of pharmaceutical companies, insurance companies, and medical schools above the needs of regular people.

At the same time, this wildly expensive system isn't even generating good outcomes. For the first time in U.S. history, life expectancy has been dropping, and we are surrounded on all sides by preventable chronic diseases like diabetes, heart disease, and even many cancers.

Confronted with this broken system, regular people are confused, disheartened, and frightened. When a simple doctor visit can cost a day's wages for many people, how can we expect people to stay on top of their self-care?

At the same time, we are subjected every day to an avalanche of healthcare information, most of it bad. Without specialized knowledge, people searching online for how they can protect their health have to wade through junk science, scammers, health ideologues, and profiteers to uncover the good information. It's no wonder people are confused about what's good for them—who can we trust when everybody seems to be yelling at the same volume?

But these challenges are not the end of the story—not even close. While there are many problems facing us, there is great hope. In fact, I believe there's much more to celebrate than there is to fear, despite the tremendous pressures and challenges we face. Thanks to innovative research and fearless healthcare providers, we are learning more and more every day about therapies that can literally reverse some of the most dreaded diseases we have today. All of that information can be a great thing as long as qualified and trusted healthcare providers help patients understand what they can trust and what they can safely ignore.

Mostly, though, I'm excited because of the patients I work with every day. I firmly believe practices like mine are the future of medicine. We are truly patient-focused. Rather than bowing to insurance companies or simply following the herd when it comes to disease treatment, we've discovered a new paradigm in medicine. And it's not complicated. We partner with patients, we take the time to educate them, and we insist on comprehensive care. It's not uncommon for our patients to remark that they've never had such personal attention or never received so much information and education.

And it's working! I've seen thousands of patients transform their lives with nothing more than the desire to be healthy and good information. It's inspiring to see that people can take their health back, they can change their lives for the better and gift themselves years of good health. The tools are there for every person in this country to break free from the tired paradigms of the past and seize control over their own health, to become truly autonomous.

All we need to do is show them the way.

TEACHER

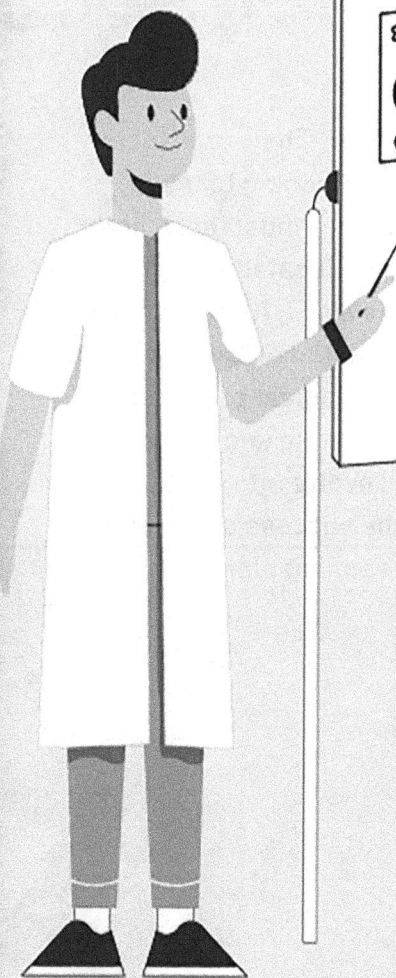
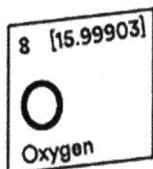
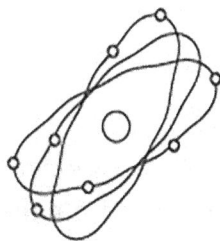
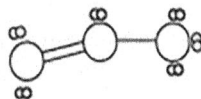

To be a good healer, one must be a teacher. The word Doctor is derived from the Latin word Docco, meaning to teach. The obligation to teach is two-fold; first they must teach both their patients and their colleagues. An educated patient is a successful patient. Not only that, it is also a fundamental and ethical right for patients to be educated on their body and their treatment choices. Second, medical providers must continue to educate each other. Sharing knowledge is the only way the field of medicine will evolve into a system that is well rounded and focused on the success of patients rather than linear, outdated treatment plans.

Conclusion

I'd like to take a moment and be earnest with you, the reader. Writing this book was quite difficult for me at times. It can be overwhelming investigating the failures facing our healthcare system. These failures I've studied while writing this book are distressing to me as a healthcare provider because this profession should be fixated on whatever can be done to help people get better. Instead, it is riddled with patients suffering- physically, emotionally, medically, and financially.

As I wrote in the last chapter, I truly am not pessimistic about the future of healthcare in the United States. I believe that our society is on the brink of a new era in human health. Medicine is going to continue to advance from our outdated reactive system and will be driven equally by technology, research, education, and most importantly compassion. These changes are not going to happen overnight, and to be realistic, will likely be unevenly distributed throughout society at first. As we enter this transitional era of medicine, it is important that the coming generations continue to push towards the future I'm invested in implementing into my clinic's today. Aside from delivering superior healthcare to everyone at a reasonable cost, it is imperative for the next generations to empower patients through education so the patient can make intelligent decisions about what is best for their care.

If it seems like there is a long way to go, that's because there is. As uncomfortable as it may be, we need to identify the problems and take them on with open eyes. As you educate yourself, there's a chance that you find yourself overwhelmed just as I was. Remember, no matter how monumental the problems appear to be, you the reader, and more importantly the patient, hold the power to influence change. Do what you can to make a difference. Vote. Tell a friend or a colleague your story. Trust your health with providers that share your ideas and not only treat you but *hear* you. Every choice you make in favor of autonomy may seem like a small step for you, but it is a giant leap forward. As word spreads, more clinic's that operate with the same mission as mine will open and more patients will be like you, insisting in being a full partner in their own care. These "small" steps will turn into a stampede that will cause the old, broken system to come crumbling down.

Always remember, you have the power, *use it*. All you need to do to create a better future is imagine it and then will it into existence, one decision at a time.

THE HIPOCRISY OF HEALTHCARE

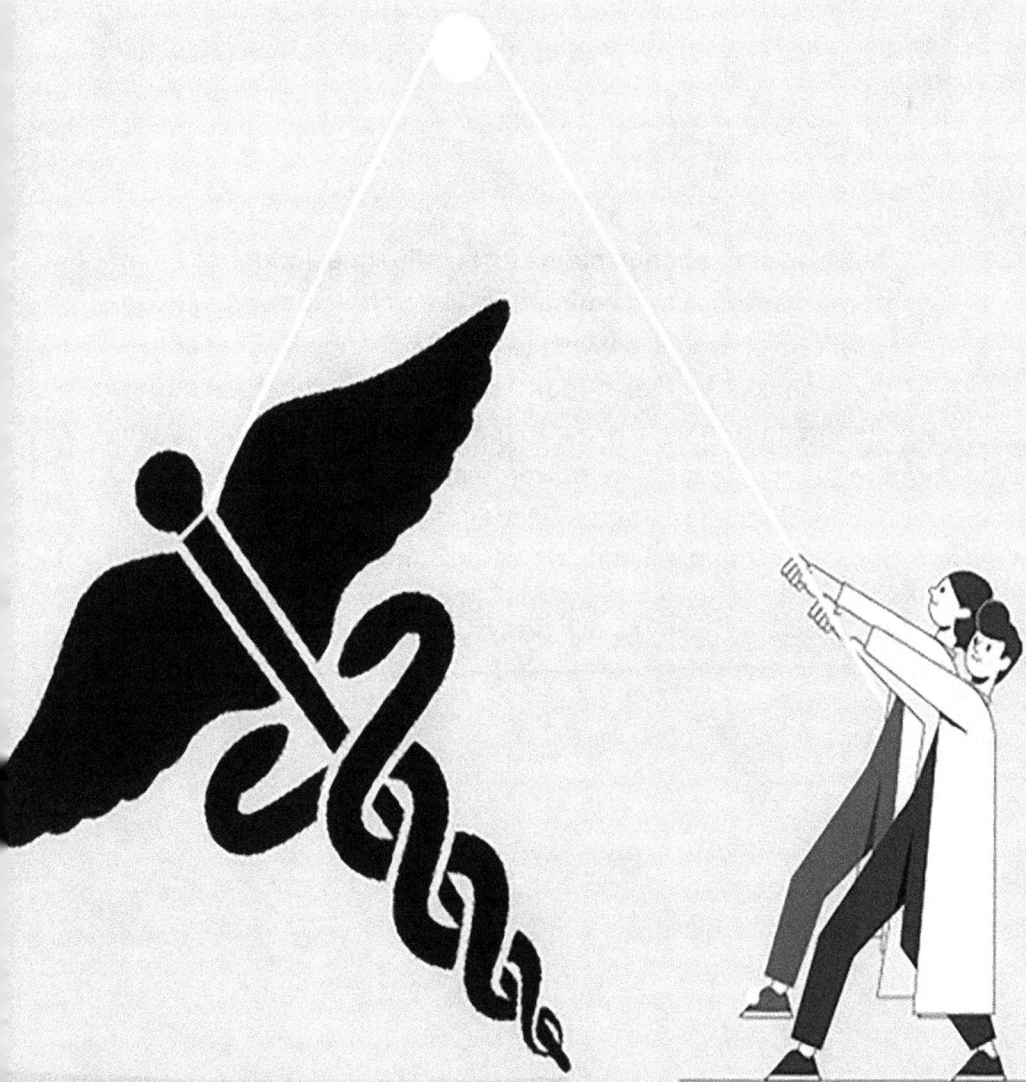

The power to change stems from influence, influence stems from awareness and education. The only way our healthcare system changes is if we the people change it. Challenge, question, ask for clarity, don't settle, we must initiate our own health autonomy in order to make the world a healthier and more fulfilled place. The power to make the wrong right is in our hands. Be the creator and leader of your own life journey and that will help others around you also.

www.ingramcontent.com/pod-product-compliance
Lightning Source LLC
Chambersburg PA
CBHW050238270326
41914CB00034BA/1966/J